Beyond Single Genes: The Role of Multiple Variants in Complex Disease

Eliot

First Printing, 2024

Table of Contents

Chapter 1: Introduction

1.1 Genetics of human traits and disease

It has long been understood that genetic variants in our DNA sequence can affect phenotype and cause disease. In the late 1980s, several seminal discoveries successfully determined genes and mutations that cause monogenic disease. In cystic fibrosis, researchers determined that a majority of cases were caused by a three base-pair deletion that affected the amino acid sequence of the chloride ion channel coded by the *CFTR* gene (Kerem et al. 1989; Rommens et al. 1989; Riordan et al. 1989). Since then, thousands of Mendelian disease genes and mutations have been discovered and many are catalogued in online databases ("OMIM - Online Mendelian Inheritance in Man" 1985; Cooper and Krawczak 1996; Landrum et al. 2014).

With the advent of microarrays and next-generation sequencing, scientists can now perform more high-throughput analyses to investigate genetic diseases caused by multiple genes as well as genetic variants with smaller individual effects. One widely applied method, the genome-wide association study (GWAS), detects genetic variants that are associated with complex traits and diseases in a large population of individuals (thousands to millions). This method arose from the "common disease, common variant" hypothesis, which argued that many common genetic diseases were caused by relatively common variants with small effect sizes and/or low penetrance (Schork et al. 2009). Thus far, GWASs have highlighted genetic loci for thousands of traits and diseases, but the majority of these variants fall into noncoding regions of the genome for which we often lack functional understanding.

Researchers have taken many approaches to elucidate the mechanisms of action of GWAS loci (Cano-Gamez and Trynka 2020) with various success stories (Smemo et al. 2014; Benjamin Joachim Schmiedel et al. 2016; D.-L. Zhu et al. 2018; Sobreira et al. 2021), but the molecular mechanisms of the vast majority of GWAS associations remains unknown. One approach which we will explore here is the association of genetic variants with an intermediate phenotype, namely gene expression levels. These expression quantitative trait loci (eQTLs) can help to elucidate functions of GWAS loci as well as offer a deeper understanding of biology and the genetic regulation of genes. We set out to review genetic variant effects and eQTLs as well as discuss some of the challenges with eQTL discovery, analysis, and association with GWAS loci.

1.2 Genetic effects on gene function and expression

1.2.1 Types of genetic variant effects

Genetic variants have various mechanisms by which they can affect gene or protein level and function, which may go on to influence complex traits and diseases. Variants may directly affect protein function, such as in the common cystic fibrosis mutation discovered in 1989: a three base pair deletion in the coding sequence of *CFTR* results in a deletion of phenylalanine in the protein's amino acid sequence, which leads to its misfolding and inability to function as a chloride ion channel in airway epithelia (Lukacs and Verkman 2012). Similarly, genetic variants may alter amino acid sequences which can, for example, disrupt binding sites or subcellular localization of the protein. In addition to altering a single amino acid residue, variants can exert more widespread effects by altering transcript and protein structure. Genetic variants in or near splice sites can alter the inclusion/exclusion of exons and introns which lead to altered transcript and protein structures, and variants can alter transcription start and end sites.

In addition to altering protein structure and function, genetic variants within transcripts can affect levels of protein or transcript via post-transcriptional regulation, such as altered transcript stability and translation rate. A common mechanism of decreased transcript stability is nonsense-mediated decay caused by variants that produce premature termination codons (also called stop-gain mutations) that fall more than 50-55 bases upstream of the 3' untranslated region of the transcript (Kurosaki, Popp, and Maquat 2019; Brandt, Gokden, et al. 2020). Premature termination codons can be produced by single nucleotide changes that create a stop codon, by frameshift mutations that alter codon sequences, or by splicing mutations that lead to frameshifts or improper transcript structure. Genetic variants in the 3' untranslated can also alter protein and RNA binding to the transcript and lead to altered degradation or localization of the transcript in the cell (Tushev et al. 2018; Vejnar et al. 2019; López-Martínez et al. 2020). These mechanisms can lead to altered transcript levels, which are detectable by RNA sequencing, or they may affect translation rate and protein levels without clear differences in mRNA abundance.

Finally, genetic variants that alter transcription rates can affect transcript and subsequently protein levels. Ultimately, transcription rate is determined by the genomic binding of and subsequent transcription by RNA polymerase II. This protein complex is directed where to bind in the genome by hundreds of proteins called transcription factors, which recognize and bind to patterns in the DNA sequence. These transcription factor binding sites may be located near the transcription start site in a region called the promoter, or up to hundreds of thousands of bases away in regions called enhancers. Genetic variants may alter transcript factor affinity for the genetic sequence, leading to altered transcription factor binding and subsequently altered chromatin accessibility, histone modifications, chromosomal looping, and/or RNA polymerase II recruitment (Kilpinen et al. 2013; McVicker et al. 2013; Kasowski et al. 2013; Waszak et al. 2015; Grubert et al. 2015). These mechanisms will lead to altered transcript levels and potentially affect protein levels and phenotype as well.

Table 1.1. Variant effects on expression, protein, and function

Primary variant effect/location	**Δ Expression level**	**Δ Protein level**	**Δ Protein structure or function**
Protein amino acid deletion/substitution	Unlikely	Unlikely	Possible
Splice site	Possible	Possible	Yes
Altered transcription start site / 5' untranslated region	Possible	Possible	Possible
Premature termination codon (>50 bases from TTS)	Yes	Yes	Possible
Premature termination codon (<50 bases from TTS)	Possible	Possible	Possible
3' untranslated region	Possible	Yes	Possible
Promoter	Yes	Yes	No
Enhancer	Yes	Yes	No

1.2.2 Expression quantitative trait loci

We can detect variants that are associated with changes in gene expression across individuals with expression quantitative trait loci, or eQTLs. Understanding these associations can offer a deeper understanding of the genetic regulation of gene expression, as well as help us explain any effects on phenotype and disease. We discover *cis*-eQTLs in large groups of individuals (tens to thousands) by comparing gene expression with genotype for all variants near the gene's transcription start site (often within one megabase) [FIG 1.1]. Multiple eVariants are tested per eGene, which may lead to multiple associated eVariants – the challenges associated with this are discussed below in *1.3.1 Statistical fine-mapping.*

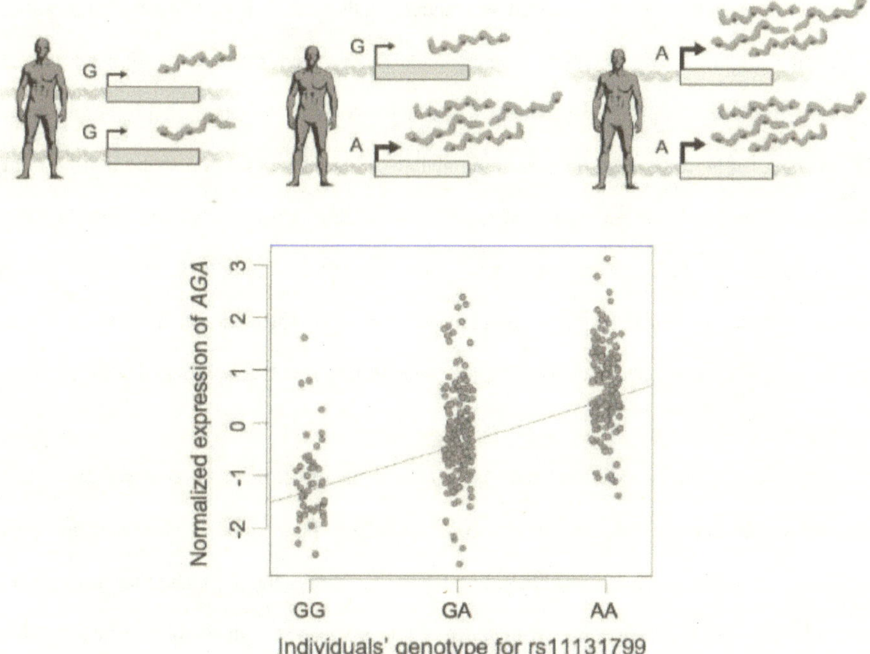

Figure 1.1. Schematic of an eQTL. (Top) Three example individuals with different genotypes for a variant that associates with altered gene expression. (Bottom) Population data for an eQTL for *AGA* gene. Individual eGene expression is plotted by individual eVariant genotype. Adapted from (Brandt and Lappalainen 2017)

We generally use linear models to discover eQTLs, by regressing normalized and log-transformed gene expression on alternative allele dosage across individuals (Ongen et al. 2016). Most eQTL studies also include covariates in the linear model to remove noise in expression measurements caused by population stratification or non-genetic sources of variation in gene expression (e.g., environmental, technical). For instance, differences in gene expression between populations could associate with every genetic variant that has different allele frequencies in the two populations. Thus, the first few principal components of the samples' genotype matrix are included as covariates in the eQTL discovery model. On the other hand, environmental conditions or technical artefacts could introduce changes in gene expression that obscure differences caused by local genetic regulation. These covariates can be known, such as sequencing run or individual sex, or they can be discovered by examining gene expression patterns across the transcriptome. One method, probabilistic estimation of expression residuals (PEER), discovers hidden factors underlying gene expression variation across individuals (Stegle et al. 2010, 2012). Known and learned factors can then be used as covariates in the eQTL linear model in order to remove confounding effects on gene expression and increase the power to discover genetic effects on gene expression.

We can quantify the magnitude of eQTLs with effect sizes. Previously, researchers reported regression coefficients learned from the eQTL linear model. However, regression coefficients have different meanings based on the unit of expression used, and they are not easily comparable across expression levels. (E.g., a variant associated with doubled gene expression could have a beta of 1 if expression doubled from 1 to 2, or 1000 if expression doubled from 1000 to 2000.) Therefore, we use the log2 allelic fold change statistic, or aFC, to interpret eQTL effects [FIG 1.2]. aFC is computed on a logarithmic scale, thus it is stable at different gene expression levels. It can be quantified using learned parameters from the eQTL linear model, or it can be determined using allele-specific expression data in individuals heterozygous for the eVariant [FIG 1.2].

$$aFC = log_2\left(\frac{ALT\ allele\ expr}{REF\ allele\ expr}\right)$$

In a population:

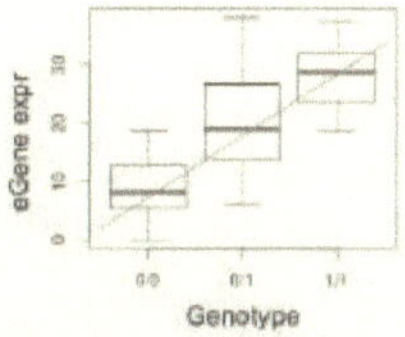

eGene expr

Genotype

$$aFC = log_2\left(\frac{E_{1/1}/2}{E_{0/0}/2}\right) = log_2\left(\frac{2 * slope}{intercept} + 1\right)$$

$$= log_2\left(\frac{2*10}{10} + 1\right) = log_2(3) = 1.6$$

In a heterozygous individual:

HAP 1 A eGene

HAP 2 G eGene

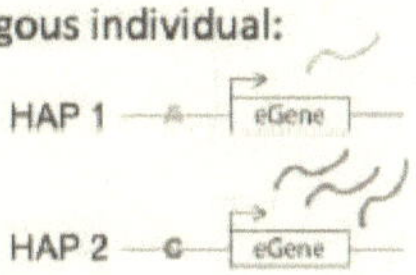

$$aFC = log_2\left(\frac{e_2}{e_1}\right) = log_2\left(\frac{3}{1}\right) = 1.6$$

Figure 1.2. Log2 allelic fold change statistic. (First row) General equation for the log allelic fold change statistics (aFC). (Second row) aFC calculation in a population. aFC is calculated using parameters from the linear model fit to the population expression and genotype data. (Third row) aFC calculation in a heterozygous individual. aFC is calculated from the number of alleles measured from each haplotype (Mohammadi et al. 2017a).

1.2.3 Other QTLs

The same methods used for eQTL discovery can be applied to a variety of molecular traits to discover other types of quantitative trait loci. From gene expression data, we can measure promoter usage (Kimura et al. 2006; Garieri et al. 2017; Alasoo et al. 2019), splicing patterns (Heinzen et al. 2008; Monlong et al. 2014), and transcript structure (Glinos et al. 2021) and determine which genetic variants are associated with differences in these measures. We can also measure protein levels to discover protein QTLs (Chick et al. 2016; Mirauta et al. 2020; B. He et al. 2020; Robins et al. 2021). Protein QTLs tend to overlap with eQTLs, with recent studies finding that 58% of protein QTLs in induced pluripotent stem cells (Mirauta et al. 2020), 59% in liver (B. He et al. 2020), and 75% in brain prefrontal cortex (Robins et al. 2021) were also eQTLs. However, the significant portion of non-overlapping protein QTLs highlight the potential role of genetic control of post-transcriptional modifications.

We can also detect QTLs for epigenomic traits, such as chromatin accessibility (Degner et al. 2012), histone modification (McVicker et al. 2013; Kasowski et al. 2013; Waszak et al. 2015; Grubert et al. 2015), or transcription factor binding (Kasowski et al. 2013; Ding et al. 2014; Waszak et al. 2015; Tehranchi et al. 2016). These epigenomic QTLs can be used to help elucidate the functional effects of eQTL variants, as is discussed in *1.3.2 Genomic Annotations*.

1.3 Determining eQTL mechanisms

1.3.1 Statistical fine-mapping

A large challenge in interpreting eQTL effects is determining which variant(s) is/are causal for the observed effect. Because of haplotype structure and linkage disequilibrium (LD) between variants, multiple variants in a region may show statistically significant associations, even if only one is causal, and the lead variant may not always be a causal variant. Adding complexity, recent massively parallel reporter assay (MPRA)-based studies have suggested that many associated loci (estimates range from 17% to 40% of tested loci) may have multiple functional variants in high LD (Abell et al. 2021; Mouri et al. 2021). Statistical fine-mapping approaches attempt to address the issues of LD by assigning a causal probability to the lead variant of the association or by narrowing the potential causal variants to a small set, though they cannot differentiate between multiple causal variants in high LD.

Statistical fine-mapping approaches often, but not always, use Bayesian statistical frameworks to estimate variants' posterior probabilities of being causal, based on the distribution of associations of all variants in a region. The causal variants identification in associated regions (CAVIAR) method jointly models association of all variants in a locus and determines variant sets at a certain posterior probability threshold, such that one can be that amount certain that the causal variant(s) lie in the variant set (Hormozdiari et al. 2014). This method improved on previous methods by allowing the modeling of multiple causal variants without the drawbacks of conditioning approaches (Hormozdiari et al. 2014). On the other hand, the causal-variant evidence mapping using nonparametric resampling (CaVEMaN) method uses a frequentist approach with resampling to estimate each variant's probability of being causal (Brown et al. 2017). Briefly, genetic and expression data are sampled with replacement, and eQTL associations are calculated for each new dataset. The assigned probability for each variant is based on the probability that it was ranked first through tenth in the resampled data (p_i), times the probability that a simulated causal variant was ranked first- through tenth-ranked variant in separate simulations (F_i): $\sum_{i=1}^{10} p_i F_i$.

Statistical fine-mapping methods may also incorporate genomic annotations to improve the prediction of causal variants. As discussed below, certain types of variants are more likely to cause changes in phenotype, so we may choose to prioritize those variants during fine-mapping. For example, the deterministic approximation of posteriors (DAP-G) method tests for the enrichment of genomic annotations among associated variants, and then re-performs associations and fine-mapping using the learned importance of the genomic annotations (Wen et al. 2016; Y. Lee et al. 2018). The enrichment of annotations in the associated variants is performed using an expectation-maximization algorithm, calculating posterior inclusion probabilities across variants with the current estimation of annotation enrichments, then fitting an updated estimation of annotation enrichments to the given annotations and resulting probabilities across variants. These estimated enrichment parameters are used to perform variant association testing, assign final posterior probabilities per variant, and determine credible sets of potentially causal variants.

1.3.2 Genomic annotations

When determining mechanisms of eQTLs, we expect to see eVariants fall into regions that can alter gene expression levels. Indeed, it has been well established that lead eQTL variants are enriched near the transcription start sites of their eGenes (Stranger et al. 2007; Lappalainen et al. 2013; GTEx Consortium 2015). eQTLs in GTEx are significantly enriched in a variety of regulatory regions from Ensembl Regulatory Build and Variant Effect Predictor, including promoters, enhancers, 5' UTR, 3' UTR, and splice sites [FIG 1.3] (Zerbino et al. 2015; McLaren et al. 2016; Cunningham et al. 2019; GTEx Consortium 2020). As expected, we also observe an enrichment of stop-gain coding and splice site variants. We additionally see an enrichment for missense and synonymous coding variants – these would be expected to alter protein function, and their direct impact on transcript level is less clear but could be caused by altered RNA binding proteins, RNA stability, or splicing patterns. The disruption of post-transcriptional regulation is certainly one mechanism that can lead to changes in gene expression but will not be the focus of this book.

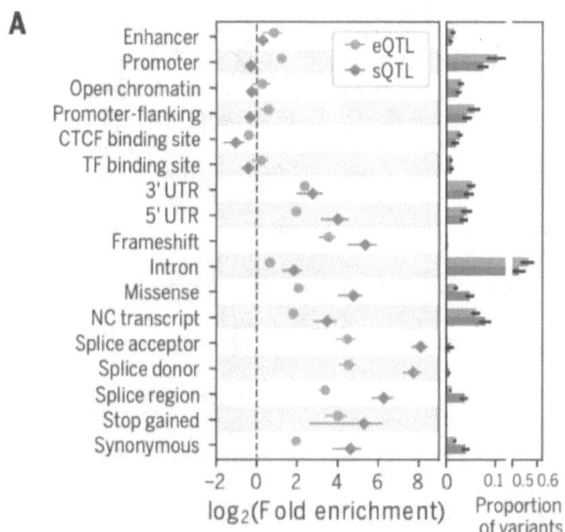

Figure 1.3. eQTL enrichment in genomic annotations. Enrichment of lead eQTL variants in various genomic annotations from Ensembl Regulatory Build and Variant Effect Predictor. Adapted from (GTEx Consortium 2020). To note, the observed lack of enrichment in "open chromatin" and "transcription factor binding sites" in GTEx eQTLs is explained by the fact that this Ensembl Regulatory Build annotation is only for sites that do not already fall into one of the other regulatory categories, thus it does not include putative transcription factor binding sites in promoters and enhancers (EMBL-EBI 2021).

As many eQTLs lie in noncoding regions of the genome, assigning function to these loci requires additional data. For example, chromatin accessibility data (DNase1 hypersensitivity sites (DHS) or ATAC-seq) (Boyle et al. 2008; Buenrostro et al. 2013) and histone modification ChIP-seq peaks (Barski et al. 2007; Heintzman et al. 2009) can highlight which regions of the genome contain accessible chromatin or are likely to bind transcription factors. Large consortium efforts have catalogued these regulatory features across a wide range of human cell types (ENCODE Project Consortium 2012; PsychENCODE Consortium 2018; Roadmap Epigenomics Consortium et al. 2015; Stunnenberg, The International Human Epigenome Consortium, and Hirst 2016). Multiple eQTL studies have investigated the overlap of lead eQTL variants with these regions, with similar results. Gaffney et al. and Lappalainen et al. both investigated eQTLs discovered in lymphoblastoid cell lines (LCLs) and discovered 4-fold and 3.4-fold enrichment in DHS open chromatin, ~2-fold and 3.5-fold enrichment in histone marks associated with active promoters, and 1.4- to 3-fold and 2.5-fold enrichment in histone marks associated with active enhancers, respectively (Gaffney et al. 2012; Lappalainen et al. 2013).

Noncoding eQTL function can be also inferred by integration with other types of QTLs. If a variant is associated with changes in gene expression and for example, chromatin accessibility, it can be inferred that the locus alters accessibility which then affects gene expression. Multiple studies have found that eQTLs, chromatin accessibility QTLs, and histone modification QTLs are often overlapping (Kasowski et al. 2013; Waszak et al. 2015; Grubert et al. 2015; McVicker et al. 2013), with one study estimating that 78% of LCL eQTL effects were mediated by chromatin activity (Waszak et al. 2015). This is compatible with GTEx eQTL genomic annotation results, which uncovered that approximately 15% of lead eQTL variants fell into 5' UTRs, 3' UTRs, coding sequence, or splice sites, leaving 85% of eQTLs with potential transcriptional regulation mechanisms [FIG 1.3] (GTEx Consortium 2020). eQTLs have been shown to have greater enrichment for transcription factor binding QTLs than other intermediate phenotype QTLs (Kilpinen et al. 2013), leading scientists to speculate that transcription factor binding may be the main mediator of regulatory genetic variant effects.

1.3.3 Transcription factor binding

Common approaches to investigate transcription factor mechanisms of eQTL effects rely on transcription factor binding information from transcription factor ChIP-seq and other experiments and predicted binding motifs. Determining overlap with transcription factor ChIP-seq peaks (Johnson et al. 2007) is straightforward, and eQTL studies observe overlap enrichment of eVariants in peaks for many transcription factors (Gaffney et al. 2012; Lappalainen et al. 2013). However, this approach provides limited information on whether the variant might directly perturb transcription factor binding. Towards this end, we can use *ex vivo* allele-specific transcription factor binding, *in vitro* low- or high-throughput transcription factor binding experiments, and transcription factor preferred binding motifs to predict if a variant will alter a transcription factor's affinity for the genetic sequence.

Several studies have experimentally investigated allelic effects of genetic variants on *ex vivo* transcription factor binding. In cases where the assayed cell line is heterozygous for an eVariant, we may be able to use allele-specific binding data to assess if either allele is preferentially bound by the transcription factor. Several efforts have catalogued allele-specific binding in individual transcription factor ChIP-seq experiments (J. Chen et al. 2016; Abramov et al. 2021). These analyses have determined thousands of common variants in the population with allelic imbalance for hundreds of specific transcription factors, but their causality cannot be assumed. Allele-specific transcription factor binding has also been assessed across individuals, discovering thousands of genetic variants associated with changes in transcription factor binding for a range of factors (Kilpinen et al. 2013; Kasowski et al. 2013; Ding et al. 2014; Waszak et al. 2015; Tehranchi et al. 2016). However, due to the high workload burden of ChIP-seq experiments, these association studies have only covered a handful of factors, mostly in relatively small sample sizes (<100 individuals). Interestingly, these studies have found limited overlap between QTL variants and transcription factor binding sites. One study of PU.1 binding found that only 33% of PU.1 QTLs mapped inside of PU.1 ChIP-seq peaks (Waszak et al. 2015), while another found that less than 1% of QTLs for five transcription factors fell into the respective transcription factor motif

(Tehranchi et al. 2016). These results suggest that *in vivo* transcription factor binding is likely coordinated between multiple factors and determining the causal transcription factor of a QTL effect may require more complex modeling.

Multiple low- and high-throughput methods can assess *in vitro* transcription factor binding affinity to genetic sequences. The electrophoretic mobility shift assay (EMSA) tests binding of transcription factors to specific DNA sequences by incubating the two together, then using gel electrophoresis to quantify transcription factor binding to the DNA sequence (Garner and Revzin 1981; Leblanc and Moss 2009). This method can identify sequences that bind transcription factors as well as quantify differences in binding between sequences, though it is low-throughput and requires hypothesized protein-DNA interactions to begin with. Systematic evolution of ligands by exponential enrichment (SELEX) performs multiple rounds of selection for protein-nucleotide binding on multiple nucleotide sequences in parallel, thus allowing more binding sites to be assayed in a single run (Tuerk and Gold 1990). SELEX-seq has also emerged as a high-throughput application of the SELEX method, capable of interrogating hundreds of thousands of DNA sequences pooled together in a single experiment (Jolma et al. 2010; Slattery et al. 2011). SELEX technologies also have the benefit of multiple rounds of data for quantification of DNA binding affinities: each round of selection represents a higher affinity of the transcription factor for the DNA sequence, which can be incorporated into biophysical models of transcription factor binding. *In vitro* interrogation cannot capture all of the complex protein-protein interactions and genomic context present in a cell's nucleus, but initial applications of SELEX-seq investigated Hox protein complexes and confirmed *ex vivo* results suggesting complex binding interactions between multiple transcription factors (Slattery et al. 2011).

Finally, transcription factor affinity for genetic sequence can be predicted *in silico* using preferred transcription factor binding motifs. Determining these motifs generally involves two steps: 1) determining which sequences a transcription factor binds to, and 2) discovering common patterns in those sequences. Transcription factor binding can be measured *ex vivo* (Kheradpour and Kellis 2014; Kulakovskiy et al. 2018; Mathelier et al. 2016) or *in vitro* (Kheradpour et al. 2013; Jolma et al. 2013; Slattery et al. 2011), and sequence affinities can be assessed by simple position weight matrices or more complex frameworks, such as biophysical models (Rastogi et al. 2018) or convolutional neural networks (Zhou and Troyanskaya 2015). Transcription factor motifs are enriched to overlap QTLs for gene expression and for intermediate phenotypes (McVicker et al. 2013; Kasowski et al. 2013; Waszak et al. 2015), solidifying the hypothesis that they are the main mediators of genetic regulatory effects on transcription.

1.3.4 Experimental approaches

In addition to using genomic annotations and transcription factor binding information to predict which eQTL variants are causal and hypothesize their mechanisms, researchers can also use experimental assays to directly profile the effects of a genetic variant on gene expression. A common method is the luciferase assay: potentially regulatory genetic sequences are inserted into a plasmid upstream of the luciferase gene, which is then added into a cell where expression is measured via the fluorescence produced when the mature luciferase enzyme degrades the added luciferin substrate (de Wet et al. 1987; Brasier, Tate, and Habener 1989). By comparing fluorescence between genetic sequences with each variant allele, we can detect expression differences caused by genetic variants.

Massively parallel reporter assays (MPRAs) also use a plasmid-based approach, inserting putative regulatory sequences into plasmids along with an arbitrary short transcript and unique reporter tags (Melnikov et al. 2012). By comparing the ratio of each tag in the expressed RNA and the plasmid DNA for thousands of regulatory sequences, researchers can determine which sequences drive expression and which genetic variants have allelic effects. MPRAs can assay tens of thousands of genetic variants at a time, which while impressive, amounts to only one or two variants tested per gene on average (Melnikov et al. 2012; Kheradpour et al. 2013; Abell et al. 2021). An even higher-throughput MPRA method, survey of regulatory elements (SuRE) reporter technology, can assess millions of sequences to determine if any produce promoter activity (van Arensbergen et al. 2019). Though all these methods measure expression in human cell nuclei with endogenous transcription factors concentrations, the regulatory sequences are present in plasmids, not their native genomic context. This means that any effects caused by local and distal sequence interactions or chromatin states cannot be assessed. To assess the effects of genetic variants in their native genomic context, we can directly edit the genomic sequence using CRISPR-Cas9 technology (Jinek et al. 2012; Ran et al. 2013). Of course, this method cannot achieve the highly parallel throughput of MPRAs, but it has the benefit of querying genetic variant effects in their native genomic context.

1.4 Context specificity of eQTLs

1.4.1 Tissues and cell types

Context specificity adds another dimension to genetic variant analysis, as many genetic variants may exert their regulatory effects in only some cell types or conditions. For instance,

GTEx eQTLs exhibit a bimodal pattern of activity across 49 surveyed tissues, where approximately a third of eQTLs are estimated to be active in all or almost all tissues, while ~20% are estimated to be active in five or fewer tissues (GTEx Consortium 2020). Multiple methods have been developed to aid researchers in determining eQTL sharing across contexts. Multiple adaptive shrinkage (mash) was used in the GTEx analysis to quantify sharing of genetic variant effects across conditions and then use those patterns to re-compute eQTL significance and effects in each tissue (Urbut et al. 2019). Another method, sn-spMF, uses matrix factorization to determine patterns of tissue-sharing and tissue-specificity (Y. He et al. 2020). When applied to GTEx eQTLs, sn-spMF learned one ubiquitous pattern, eight patterns that represent multiple tissues but not all, and 14 patterns that represent a single tissue. They found that 20% of tested eQTLs matched the ubiquitous pattern, while 53% matched a tissue-specific pattern – ~12% matched both. Interestingly, eQTLs that were active across tissues were enriched for more transcription factors in promoters than enhancers, while tissue-specific eQTLs showed the opposite pattern (Y. He et al. 2020). Complicating matters farther, some eQTLs appear to have opposite directional effects in different tissues, suggesting the presence of multiple causal variants in the locus and/or distinct gene regulation mechanisms between tissues (Mizuno and Okada 2019).

However, most tissues are heterogeneous compositions of multiple cell types, complicating interpretation of tissue eQTLs. Studies have investigated eQTLs in patient-derived cell lines, especially lymphoblastoid cell lines, fibroblasts, and induced pluripotent stem cells (Gaffney et al. 2012; Lappalainen et al. 2013; Gutierrez-Arcelus et al. 2015; GTEx Consortium 2015). However, cell lines cannot recapitulate all cell types observed *in vivo*, and they may be unstable, especially after many passages (Oh et al. 2013). Alternatively, cell types can be sorted from heterogeneous patient tissue samples. This approach has been mainly applied for blood and immune cell eQTLs

(Fairfax et al. 2012; Raj et al. 2014; Naranbhai et al. 2015; Kasela et al. 2017; Kim-Hellmuth et al. 2017), notably by the BLUEPRINT epigenome project and the Database of Immune Cell Expression, eQTLs, and Epigenomics (DICE) that have assayed eQTLs in a variety of blood and immune cell types (L. Chen et al. 2016; Benjamin J. Schmiedel et al. 2018; Chandra et al. 2021). However, cell sorting and isolation from other tissues are time and cost intensive, and in some cases cell sorting may be impossible if, for example, cell surface markers are not known. Thus, these methods have not been widely applied to other cell types (T. Zhang et al. 2018; Young et al. 2021). Recently, single cell sequencing has also been applied to discover cell type eQTLs in cell lines (Sarkar et al. 2019; Cuomo et al. 2020; Jerber et al. 2021; Neavin et al. 2021) and blood and immune cells (van der Wijst et al. 2018), though future efforts should be able to apply single cell sequencing to additional tissues to discover eQTLs for adequately abundant cell types (Mandric et al. 2020).

Cell type specificity of eQTLs can also be inferred from tissue bulk sequencing data *in silico*. Briefly, cell type composition estimates are calculated based on sample gene expression, and these estimates can be included in an interaction model of genotype and cell type composition on gene expression:

$$E \sim u + \beta_G * G + \beta_C * C + \beta_{GxC} * G * C + cov$$

where E is eGene expression, G is eVariant genotype, and C is cell type composition estimate. The β_{GxC} term represents the interaction of cell type and genotype on gene expression and when significantly different from zero, implies that allelic effects differ between cell types. These methods may use a set of marker genes (Westra et al. 2015; Patel et al. 2021) or more complex algorithms (Aran, Hu, and Butte 2017; Kim-Hellmuth et al. 2020; Aguirre-Gamboa et al. 2020; Park et al. 2021) to estimate a cell type's abundance in gene expression data. Kim-Hellmuth et al.

discovered cell-type-interacting eQTLs in GTEx tissues using seven cell type estimates from XCell (Aran, Hu, and Butte 2017; Kim-Hellmuth et al. 2020). Interestingly, cell-type-interacting eQTLs were more tissue-specific than general eQTLs, as well as being predictive of the original eQTL for the eGene being tissue-specific (Kim-Hellmuth et al. 2020).

1.4.2 Environmental conditions and immune stimulation

eQTL effects may also vary within the same cell type across environmental conditions. eQTL activity in various conditions can be investigated to discover context-specific and context-variable eQTL effects, including clinical phenotypes (Knowles et al. 2017; Taylor et al. 2018) and *in vitro* treatments (Maranville et al. 2011; Smirnov et al. 2012; Kariuki et al. 2016; Moyerbrailean et al. 2016; Knowles et al. 2018; Findley et al. 2019, 2021). These approaches may detect eQTLs and then compare between conditions, or they may use genotype-environment interaction models to discover eQTLs that vary across contexts. One major advance for the discovery of gene-by-environment interactions on gene expression was the use of allele-specific expression data. Since allele-specific expression is measured within an individual, confounding genetic background and environmental effects are controlled for.

Many studies have investigated immune response eQTLs, or those whose effects change when immune or immune-responsive cells are treated with viral (M. N. Lee et al. 2014; Randolph et al. 2020), microbial (Barreiro et al. 2012; M. N. Lee et al. 2014; Fairfax et al. 2014; Kim et al. 2014; Kim-Hellmuth et al. 2017; Alasoo et al. 2018; Brandt, Kim-Hellmuth, et al. 2020; Nédélec et al. 2016), signaling (M. N. Lee et al. 2014; Fairfax et al. 2014; Alasoo et al. 2018), or other stimuli. These studies have found many eQTLs that are not detectable at baseline, non-stimulated conditions, highlighting the importance of context specificity in eQTL effects. Many of these effects have also been shown to be time-dependent: for instance, Kim-Hellmuth et al. measured gene expression at three timepoints and discovered activating and suppressive immune response eQTLs with early transient, late, and prolonged effects (Kim-Hellmuth et al. 2017). They found that prolonged immune response eQTLs tended to show congruent gene expression (i.e., higher gene expression at the time points with a significant eQTL), whereas early transient and late immune response eQTLs were split between congruent and non-congruent gene expression, suggesting that higher gene expression was not directly driving the observed eQTL. Similarly, Gutierrez-Arcelus et al. investigated allelic gene expression across eight time points of memory CD4+ T cell stimulation and found examples of both positive and negative correlation between gene expression and allelic imbalance (Gutierrez-Arcelus et al. 2020). These results suggest that context-specific genetic effects on gene expression involve complex regulation and cannot be explained by binary gene expression effects.

1.5 Interpreting GWAS loci

Determining molecular mechanisms of GWAS loci faces many of the same challenges as eQTLs, namely fine-mapping, functional effects, and context specificity. eQTLs can be used to understand one layer of the GWAS loci's molecular mechanism, as we can infer that the genetic effect on a GWAS trait is mediated by an eGene's expression if the GWAS trait and eQTL share a genetic signal. Colocalization approaches determine whether GWAS and eQTL signals are consistent with (a) shared causal variant(s), or if they are more likely to be caused by separate signals. These approaches generally examine all possible causal variant configurations in a given region and determine their posterior probabilities based on GWAS and eQTL summary statistics as well as prior signal sharing estimates (Giambartolomei et al. 2014; Hormozdiari et al. 2016).

The ENLOC method additionally estimates prior signal sharing probability from the genome-wide enrichment of eQTLs in GWAS loci (Wen, Pique-Regi, and Luca 2017), which offers a solution for the practical problems with prior selection when using the coloc method (Wallace 2020).

Colocalization has led to candidate molecular mechanisms of many GWAS loci, especially when combined with experimental and functional information. For instance, Barbeira et al. investigated the colocalization of 87 GWAS traits with GTEx eQTLs and splicing QTLs and identified target genes for 47% of investigated GWAS loci (Barbeira et al. 2021). However, due to pleiotropy, a single GWAS locus may colocalize with eQTLs for multiple genes, complicating interpretation of the relevant molecular mechanisms. Additionally, even with eQTLs and splicing QTLs measured in 49 tissues, 53% of GWAS loci remained without a colocalized signal (Barbeira et al. 2021), perhaps highlighting the need for eQTLs in a wider variety of contexts or suggesting that many GWAS loci have molecular mechanisms that do not involve transcriptional regulation. On the first point, cell-type interacting eQTLs have been shown to colocalize with GWAS loci in cases where tissue-wide eQTLs do not (Kim-Hellmuth et al. 2020), and gene-by-environment interactions are enriched for target GWAS genes (Moyerbrailean et al. 2016; Findley et al. 2021). These results suggest that understanding genetic regulation in additional contexts may be an important key to elucidating functions of GWAS loci.

Chapter 2: Gene expression and genetic regulation across tissues[1]

2.1 Introduction

High-throughput sequencing has enabled the study of genetics and gene expression across large populations of individuals. Microarrays and exome sequencing have given way to genome sequencing, allowing researchers to investigate the extensive noncoding regions of the genome, while RNA sequencing allows for the study of gene expression across tissues and environmental conditions. Using these data, two important methods have arisen to link genetic variation in the population with phenotype. Expression quantitative trait loci (eQTLs) associate variants with changes in gene expression in specific tissues or conditions, while genome wide association studies (GWASs) associate genetic variants in the human population with changes in disease risk or phenotype.

Recently, the Genotype Tissue Expression (GTEx) Consortium has identified thousands of *cis*-eQTLs in the human population that affect gene expression across 49 tissues (GTEx Consortium 2015, 2020; GTEx Consortium et al. 2017). These variants are enriched in *cis*-regulatory elements (CREs) such as promoters and enhancers, implying that many eQTLs impact gene regulation via non-coding mechanisms. We observe that GTEx eQTLs exhibit a bimodal

---

[1] Portions of this chapter are adapted from GTEx Consortium. (2020). The GTEx Consortium atlas of genetic regulatory effects across human tissues. *Science*. 2020;369: 1318–1330.

Genetic, gene expression, eQTL, fine-mapping, and GWAS colocalization data used in these analyses were provided by the GTEx Consortium. Pejman Mohammadi performed the non-monotonic cross-tissue model fitting. All remaining analyses were performed by Elise Flynn.

pattern of activity across the 49 surveyed tissues, where over a third of eQTLs are estimated to be active in all or almost all tissues, while another third are estimated to be active in five or fewer tissues (GTEx Consortium 2020). Though this large portion of eQTLs are ubiquitously active, they may display variable effect sizes across tissues; the reasons for this variability have not yet been investigated.

Similarly to eQTLs, many discovered GWAS loci lie in noncoding regions of the genome. However, adding another layer of complexity to the interpretation of GWAS loci, the causal tissues and cell types of complex diseases and traits are not always known (Cano-Gamez and Trynka 2020). While biological and medical research of specific diseases can shed light on the causal tissues of the disease etiology, we can also use colocalization with eQTLs to pinpoint cell types and conditions where the genetic variants may be regulating gene expression. This can help determine the biological mechanisms by which genetic variants affect gene expression and subsequent disease risk.

In this chapter, we investigate cross-tissue patterns of eQTLs and gene expression in the GTEx v8 dataset (GTEx Consortium 2020). First, we determined how eQTL effect size and eGene expression are related across tissues, finding cases of both increasing and decreasing correlations between the two measures. Next, we discovered non-monotonic relationships between eQTL effect size and eGene expression, highlighting several examples. Finally, we investigated GWAS genes to determine if putative causal tissues show specific patterns of gene expression or eQTL effects, observing higher magnitudes of both measurements in relevant tissues. These analyses highlight the complex relationships between eQTL effects and gene expression across tissues, emphasizing the need for further research into the tissue specificity of regulatory variant effects.

2.2 Materials and Methods

2.2.1 Allelic fold change calculation

We used the log2 allelic fold change statistic (aFC) to quantify variant effects on gene expression (Mohammadi et al. 2017b). This measurement should be stable across gene expression levels and is calculated from population-level data with the basic formula:

$$aFC = log_2\left(\frac{\beta_1}{\beta_o} + 1\right) \qquad \text{(Eq 2.1)}$$

where β_1 is the slope and β_0 is the intercept of a linear model fit to the gene expression and alternative allele dosage across individuals. For this analysis, we did not include tissue-specific covariates in the linear model.

We chose to focus our analyses on one "top" eVariant per eGene across tissues. For each eGene, we looked at significant eQTLs across all tissues and selected the eVariant with the largest aFC effect size. This eVariant became known as the "top eVariant," and the tissue that it was found in (that with the largest significant effect size) was called the "discovery tissue." For each top eVariant, we calculated an effect size for the effect of that eVariant on eGene expression in each GTEx tissue. To enable discovery of cross-tissue patterns, we only included eQTLs where at least half of the GTEx tissues had median expression greater than zero TPM in further analysis.

2.2.2 Cross-tissue aFC and expression correlation

To examine if there were relationships between eQTL effect size and eGene expression level, we performed cross-tissue Spearman correlations. For each top eVariant, we correlated tissue aFC with eGene median transcripts per million (TPM) for all tissues that had a median TPM greater than zero. In order to make the sign of the correlation coefficient interpretable for both positive and negative effect size eQTLs, we flipped the sign of the effect sizes (multiplied by −1) if the discovery tissue eQTL effect size was negative. This ensured that the discovery effect size was always labeled as positive and correlations could be interpreted the same way for both positive and negative effect size eQTLs.

To keep our analysis straightforward, we chose to focus on eQTLs where most tissues showed effects in the same direction. Thus, we filtered out eQTL correlations that had "unclear" directions based on any of the following conditions: 1) over half of the tissue effect sizes were in the opposite direction of the discovery tissue effect; 2) any tissue effect size was in the opposite direction of the discovery tissue effect and had a magnitude of at least half the discovery tissue magnitude; or 3) the discovery effect size was 6.64 or higher, which is the maximum possible calculated aFC and often corresponds to eQTLs with low allele frequency and unstable effect sizes [FIG 2.1C]. By filtering "unclear" direction correlations and transforming effect sizes such that the discovery tissue effect was always positive, positive correlations could be interpreted as an increase in effect size magnitude with increasing eGene expression [FIG 2.1B], and negative correlations could be interpreted as a decrease in effect size magnitude with increasing eGene expression [FIG 2.1A].

2.2.3 Non-monotonic cross-tissue models

We next examined non-monotonic relationships between eQTL effect size and eGene expression across tissues. We fit flat (M0), linear (M1), and normal bell-curve (M2) models across tissues to quantile-normalized eQTL aFC effect sizes and log10 median eGene TPM for our top eQTLs. The M0 model was based on the average eQTL aFC across tissues, and the M1 model was based on a linear regression of aFC vs. $\log_{10}$(TPM) values across tissues. The M2 model was fit using a non-linear least squares method for a scaled version of the normal distribution probability density function:

$$f(x) = a * \frac{1}{\sigma\sqrt{2\Pi}} e^{-\frac{1}{2}\left(\frac{x-\mu}{\sigma}\right)^2} + b \qquad \text{(Eq 2.2)}$$

resulting in *mu* (***μ***), *sigma* (***σ***), scale (*a*), and intercept (*b*) parameters.

The optimal model was chosen using Bayesian information criteria (BIC). This method balances the fact that the addition of parameters can lead to overfitting by penalizing the number of parameters versus the resulting residuals. We calculated BIC for each model with the following equation:

$$BIC = n * ln(var(r, 1)) + k * ln(n) \qquad \text{(Eq 2.3)}$$

where *n* was the number of datapoints, *r* was the residuals of real data from the model, and *k* was the number of parameters fit by each model.

The best model was chosen in a stepwise fashion. If M2 had the lowest BIC, its significance was tested by finding the standard deviation of 20 bootstrapped M2 BIC calculations, then dividing the differences between M2/M0 and M2/M1 by this standard deviation. If the standardized differences versus both M0 and M1 were greater than one, M2 was chosen as the best model. If those criteria were not achieved and M1 was lower than M0, the significance of M1 vs M0 was tested in a similar manner: dividing the difference in BICs by the standard deviation of M1 BIC based on bootstrapping and requiring that number to be greater than one. In all other cases, M0 was chosen as the best model.

2.2.4 Allele-specific expression analysis

For eQTLs that were determined to fit the M2 model, we examined individual allele-specific expression (ASE) effect sizes to confirm the observed eQTL effect patterns. ASE can be calculated in heterozygous individual using the general equation:

$$ASE\ aFC = log_2\left(\frac{E_A+c}{E_R+c}\right) \quad \text{(Eq 2.4)}$$

where E_A/E_R is measured expression of the alternative and reference alleles, respectively, and c is the pseudocount value to account for cases of mono-allelic expression. ASE hypothetically controls for many confounding factors, since expression of each allele is measured in the same individual. For our ASE calculations, we used RNA-seq reads aligned with allele-specific correction by WASP (van de Geijn et al. 2015). Individual genotypes were phased using population-based and read-backed phasing with Phaser, which allowed us to phase eQTL variants with expressed coding variant genotypes and calqculate ASE for each selected eQTL variant and associated gene (Castel et al. 2016). We used a pseudocount of one and included samples heterozygous for the eQTL variant where at least twenty RNA-seq reads aligned to a phased and measurable coding variant. We then calculated the median ASE per tissue across all individuals heterozygous for the eQTL variant. We included tissues with at least ten individuals in our further analyses, including visual examination of cross-tissue relationships between eQTL ASE effect size and $\log_{10}$(eGene TPM) expression.

We next examined within-tissue eQTL ASE-based effect sizes across individuals within each tissue. Our motivation was to determine if within-tissue slopes fit the cross-tissue pattern we observed, such that tissues at the rising side of the bell curve should have positive slopes, while tissues on the falling side should have negative slopes. We used two approaches to determine within tissue slopes, one parametric and one non-parametric. For our parametric method, we fit a linear model to ASE effect sizes versus $\log_{10}$(eGene TPM) per tissue across all individuals with at least ten reads aligned to the coding SNP. For our non-parametric method, we determined the median ASE of the lower and higher halves of individuals based on $\log_{10}$(eGene TPM), as well as the median $\log_{10}$(eGene TPM) of each half. We then calculated the line between the two median points. For each method, we then compared the calculated slopes across tissues to determine if tissues on the rising and falling sides had positive and negative slopes, respectively. We formalized this comparison with a Wilcoxon rank sum test of the two sets of slopes.

2.2.5 eGene and eVariant properties

To get a deeper understanding of expression-correlated eQTLs, we examined properties of their associated eGenes and eVariants. We fine-mapped all top eQTLs and selected those that had a single top CaVEMaN fine-mapped eVariant (Brown et al. 2017). We gathered information on median eGene TPM, median eQTL effect size, and the eVariant's GTEx minor allele frequency across tissues for each top eQTL, and we compared these statistics between correlated and non-correlated eQTLs using Wilcoxon rank sum tests. We then overlapped the fine-mapped eVariants with transcription factor ChIP-seq peaks and DNase-seq peaks from Ensembl Regulatory Build v91 (Cunningham et al. 2019). We compared overlaps between fine-mapped eVariants for correlated and non-correlated eQTLs using Fisher's exact tests and Wilcoxon rank sum tests.

2.2.6 Determining GWAS genes

In order to study the cross-tissue eQTL effect size and eGene expression patterns in GWAS loci, we linked genes to GWAS loci using colocalization and nearest gene methods. Colocalization between GWAS loci and GTEx tissue eQTLs was performed using ENLOC, with colocalization defined by a regional conditional probability greater (rcp) than 0.5 (Barbeira et al. 2021; Wen, Pique-Regi, and Luca 2017). For each colocalized GWAS/eQTL locus, we determined the nearest protein-coding or lncRNA gene based on absolute distance of the lead colocalizing variant to a gene's transcription start site (TSS). Because GWAS signals were colocalized with eQTLs from all 49 tissues, many colocalized eGenes and nearest genes appeared multiple times for the same GWAS trait with different lead SNPs. In order to remove this redundancy, we removed duplicated colocalized genes and nearest genes for each GWAS trait by first choosing one colocalized eGene with the highest rcp per each nearest gene-GWAS trait pair, and then choosing one nearest gene with the closest TSS per each colocalized eGene-GWAS trait pair. This resulted in two gene sets, 1,110 colocalized eGenes and 1,096 nearest genes, with each gene associated with one or more GWAS traits. The union of these gene sets is referred to as GWAS genes.

2.2.7 Properties of GWAS genes

We next explored the tissue properties of colocalized and nearest GWAS genes, with the hypothesis that tissues with a potential causal role in disease should be enriched for high eQTL effect size, high gene expression, or both. In order to achieve a fair comparison of tissues that differ in their overall expression profiles or regulatory effects, we used an additional genome-wide background set of tissue expression and eQTL effects in all protein-coding and lincRNA genes.

First, we determined the tissue with the highest significant eQTL effect size (absolute aFC) and the tissue with the maximum median expression (transcripts per million, TPM) for each gene in the GWAS gene sets and the background gene set. Next, we analyzed properties of GWAS genes in GWAS-trait-relevant tissues. We calculated tissue aFC and expression ranks of tissue *t* for gene *i* using rank statistics:

aFC rank statistic: $r_{it} = \text{rank}(|a_{it}| \text{ in } |Ai|)/Ni$

expression rank statistic: $r_{it} = \text{rank}(e_{it} \text{ in } Ei)/Ni$

These were intended to normalize ranks based on *N*, the number of tissues that were not NA for the given measurement. Tissues that had a median TPM of 0 were assigned an expression rank statistic of 1/*N*; all other expression and aFC measurements were assigned a rank statistic of rank/*N*, with a higher rank statistic corresponding to a higher relative aFC or expression level. aFC rank statistics were calculated for the top eVariant for the eGene, as described in *Allelic fold change calculation.*

For a subset of GWAS traits with less ambiguous tissue of origin, we assigned a tissue group (blood, brain, immune, or metabolic) to the trait, and we then performed literature research to select hypothesized trait-relevant tissues for each trait [TABLE 2.1]. We examined the distributions of aFC and expression rank statistics for trait-relevant tissues for colocalized eGenes and nearest genes, with the hypothesis that an eQTL should have high effect size or eGene expression in tissues relevant to causal disease mechanisms. To account for the tissue-specific aFC and gene expression patterns (e.g. blood has low expression levels for most genes), we performed paired Wilcoxon signed-rank tests between trait-relevant tissue rank statistics for colocalized and nearest genes and tissue-specific null rank statistics (the median rank statistic of a given tissue in our background gene set).

2.3 Results

2.3.1 Cross-tissue correlation of eQTL effects and eGene expression

We set out to determine if eQTL effect sizes across tissues correlated with eGene expression. Of those eQTLs where at least half of the GTEx tissues had a non-zero median eGene expression, eQTL effect size and eGene expression level were significantly correlated across tissues for 2,637 top eQTLs (5% Benjamini-Hochberg FDR; N=26,499) (FIG 2.1D). Of these, 666 are filtered out because of an unclear correlation direction. The remaining correlations are split among positive correlations with a positive discovery tissue effect size (n=400), positive correlations with a negative discovery tissue effect size (n=634), negative correlations with a positive discovery tissue effect size (n=526), and negative correlations with a negative discovery tissue effect size (n=411) (FIG 2.1D). The sign of the discovery tissue effect size represents whether the alternative allele of the eVariant is associated with an increase or decrease in eGene expression. Positive correlations represent increasing effect size magnitude with increasing eGene expression, and negative correlations represent decreasing effect size magnitude with increasing eGene expression. These findings demonstrate that regulation of eQTL effects is complex and cannot be explained by straightforward on versus off expression-based mechanisms.

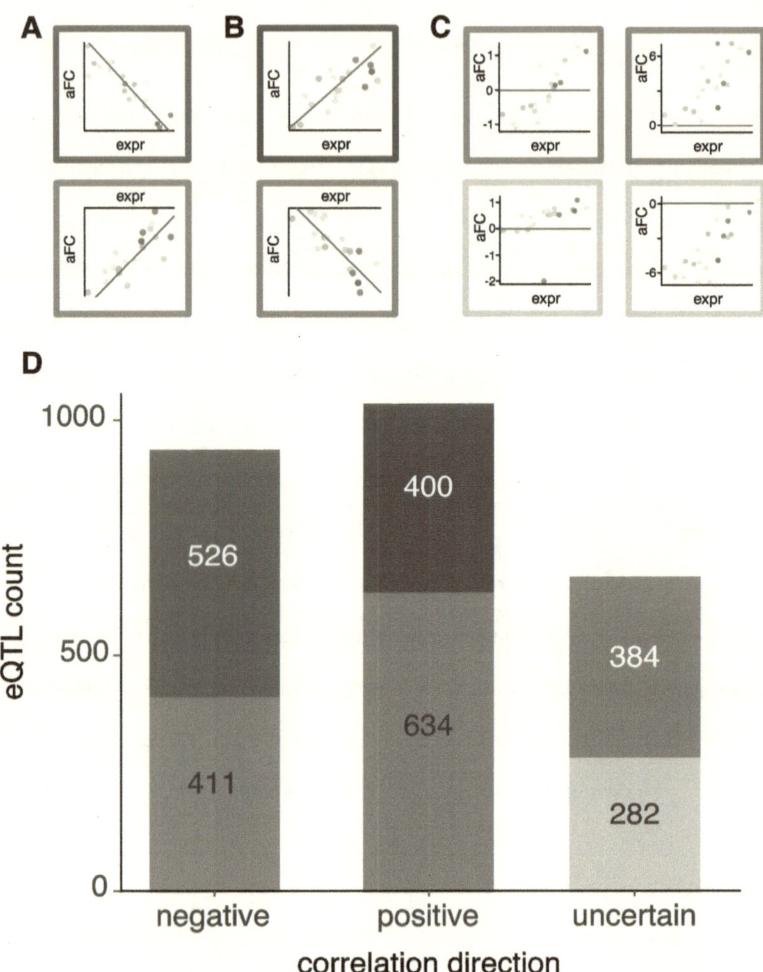

Figure 2.1: Cross-tissue eGene expression-eQTL effect correlations. A-C) Cartoon examples of negative (A), positive (B), and uncertain (C) correlation directions are shown. Each dot is a tissue and eQTL effect size is plotted versus median eGene expression. **D)** Top eQTLs with a significant correlation between eQTL effect size and median cis-eGene expression across tissues (5% Benjamini-Hochberg FDR; N=26,499).

2.3.2 Properties of expression-correlated eQTLs

Next, we examined gene and variant properties of expression-correlated eQTLs. We found that correlated eQTLs had higher eGene expression than non-correlated eQTLs (difference = 0.43 TPM, Wilcoxon $p = 1.6x10^{-13}$) [FIG 2.2A,D]. This could potentially be explained by the expression levels needed to detect accurate eQTL effects across multiple tissues: if a gene is very lowly expressed across tissues, we would have limited power to detect changes in expression or eQTL effects. However, we also found that negatively correlated eQTLs had higher eGene expression than positively correlated eQTLs (median difference = 2.95 TPM, Wilcoxon $p = 1.3x10^{-130}$) [FIG 2.2A,D]. This pattern suggests that eQTL activity may tend to increase and then decrease as eGene expression increases.

We then examined properties of fine-mapped eQTL variants and found that correlated eQTLs had eVariants with higher absolute median effect sizes and higher minor allele frequencies (MAF) than non-correlated eQTLs (differences = 0.11 aFC, 0.07 MAF, Wilcoxon ps = $7.6x10^{-294}$, $4.4x10^{-87}$, respectively) [FIG 2.2B,C,D]. Similarly to our findings of higher eGene expression in correlated eQTLs, this could be related to power issues of detecting changes in eQTL effects across tissues. We also found that positively correlated eVariants had larger effect sizes and were more common than negatively correlated eVariants (differences = 0.05 aFC, 0.05 MAF, Wilcoxon ps = $2.7x10^{-12}$, $2.7x10^{-15}$) [FIG2.2B,C,D].

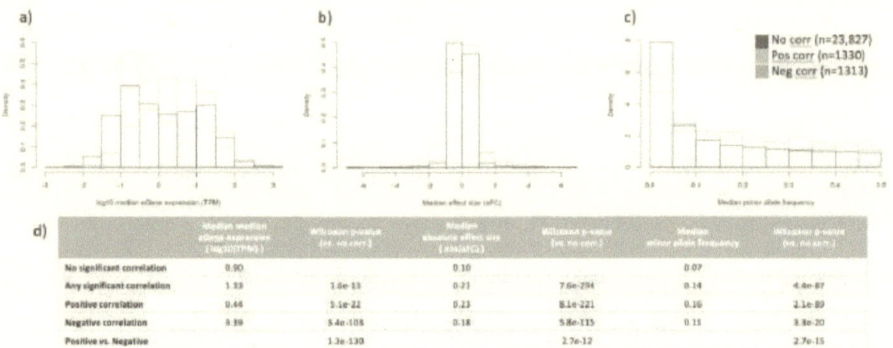

	Median median eGene expression (log10(TPM))	Wilcoxon p-value (vs. no corr.)	Median absolute effect size (abs(aFC))	Wilcoxon p-value (vs. no corr.)	Median minor allele frequency	Wilcoxon p-value (vs. no corr.)
No significant correlation	0.90		0.10		0.07	
Any significant correlation	1.33	1.6e-13	0.21	7.6e-294	0.14	4.4e-87
Positive correlation	0.44	5.1e-22	0.23	8.1e-221	0.16	2.1e-89
Negative correlation	3.39	5.4e-108	0.18	5.8e-115	0.11	3.3e-20
Positive vs. Negative		1.3e-130		2.7e-12		2.7e-15

Figure 2.2: eGene, eQTL, and eVariant features of cross-tissue correlated and uncorrelated eQTLs. **A)** Histogram of the median of median per-tissue eGene expression across tissues with greater than 0 TPM per eQTL gene. **B)** Histogram of median effect size across tissues per eQTL. **C)** Histogram of median minor allele frequency across tissues per eQTL variant. **D)** Summary statistics table of medians and Wilcoxon rank sum tests between correlation types for the listed eQTL features. Wilcoxon tests were run vs. eQTLs with no significant correlation, except for the last row of tests of positively-correlated eQTLs vs. negatively-correlated eQTLs.

We next looked at transcription factor binding and chromatin accessibility annotations to understand the mechanisms and context variability of correlated eQTLs. We found that significantly correlated eQTLs were enriched for transcription factor ChIP-seq and DNase I hypersensitivity site (DHS) peaks compared to non-significant eQTLs (TFBS OR = 1.69, Fisher's $p = 5.0x10^{-15}$; DHS OR = 1.57, Fisher's $p=3.0x10^{-11}$) [FIG 2.3A]. When correlated eQTLs were split by direction, negatively correlated eQTLs had higher enrichment than positively correlated eQTLs (TFBS ORs = 2.06, 1.31, Fisher's ps = $1.9x10^{-15}$, $4.6x10^{-3}$; DHS ORs = 2.07, 1.57, Fisher's ps = $8.2x10^{-16}$, 0.29, for negative and positive direction eQTLs, respectively). Out of all eQTLs that overlapped at least one TFBS or DHS, significantly correlated eQTLs overlapped sites in more ENCODE cell types/tissues than non-significantly correlated eQTLs (Wilcoxon ps = $5.2x10^{-3}$, $2.1x10^{-4}$) [FIG 2.3B], implying that surrounding regions of correlated eQTLs are accessible in more cell types than non-correlated eQTLs.

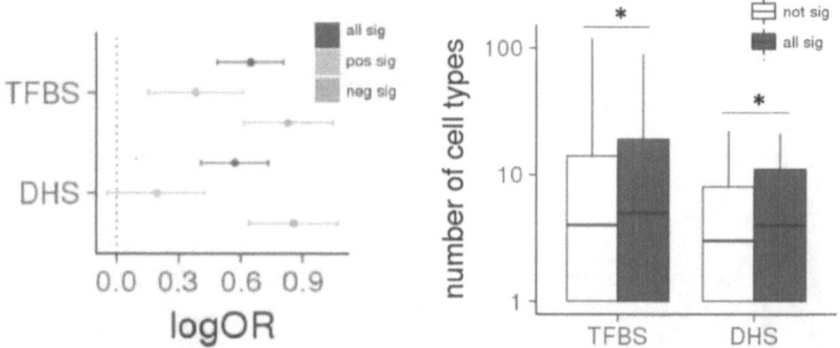

Figure 2.3: TF binding of cross-tissue correlated and uncorrelated eQTLs. **Left)** We examined annotations of fine-mapped eQTLs that had a single top CaVEMaN finemapped variant (e.g. no perfect linkage). Significantly correlated eQTLs were enriched for TFBS and DHS compared to non-significant eQTLs (TFBS OR=1.6, Fisher's p=7.2e-15; DNase OR=1.3, Fisher's p=6.5e-12). Negatively-correlated eQTLs were more significantly enriched than positively-correlated eQTLs. **Right)** Out of all eQTLs that overlapped at least one TFBS or DHS, significantly correlated eQTLs overlapped sites in more ENCODE cell types/tissues than non-significantly correlated eQTLs (Wilcoxon p=5.2e-3, 2.1e-4), implying that surrounding regions of correlated eQTLs are accessible in more cell types than non-significantly correlated eQTLs.

2.3.3 Non-monotonic relationships of eQTL effects and eGene expression

Given that we discovered eQTLs with both increasing and decreasing effects with increasing eGene expression, we next investigated if any eQTLs had non-monotonic relationships with eGene expression. To do this, we fit flat, linear, and bell-curve models to normalized eQTL aFCs and $\log_{10}$(eGene TPMs) across tissues for our top eQTLs. We found 1,043 eQTLs that best fit the linear model and 233 eQTLs that best fit the bell-curve model of the three models, based on Bayesian information criteria [FIG 2.4]. We found that 95.8% of linear eQTLs and 68.7% of bell curve eQTLs were also discovered by correlation, though 31.3% of bell curve eQTLs were not previously discovered.

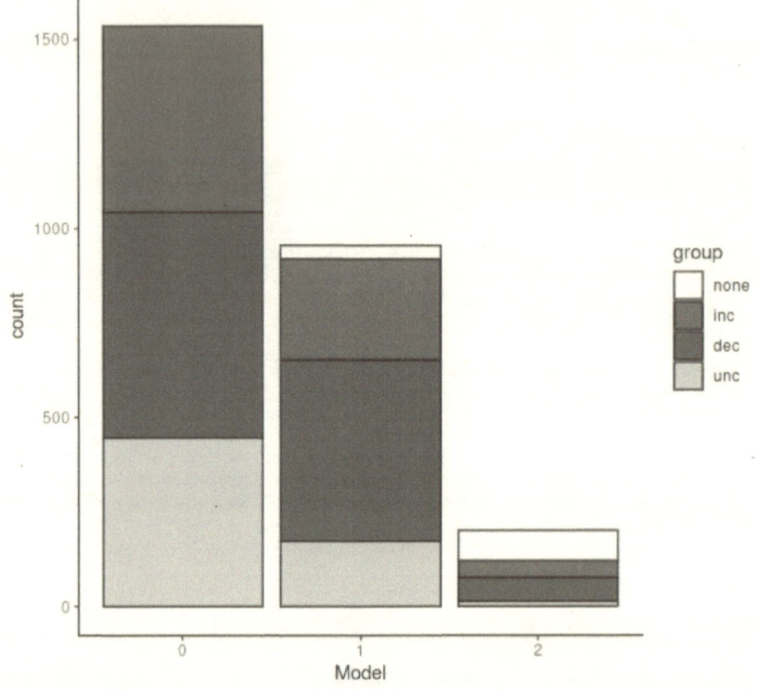

Figure 2.4: Non-monotonic model of cross-tissue eGene expression-eQTL effect. Top eQTLs plotted by best model. Bars are colored by their Spearman correlation status/direction. 1,043 eQTLs best fit the linear model (1) and 233 eQTLs that best fit the bell-curve model (2). 22,249 eQTLs that fit model 0 and were not significant in the Spearman correlation analysis are not shown.

We next examined eGene and eQTL properties of linear and bell curve eQTLs. Similarly to our analysis of correlated eQTLs, we found that linear eQTLs had higher effect sizes and higher minor allele frequencies than eQTLs that fit neither model [FIG 2.5]. Interestingly, bell curve eQTLs had even higher effect sizes and minor allele frequencies. We also observed that linear eQTLs had lower eGene expression than eQTLs that fit neither model, while bell curve eQTLs had even lower eGene expression [FIG 2.5]. While the effect size and allele frequency findings could be explained by increasing magnitudes needed to discover variability with each more complex model, the decreased expression levels do not have a clear explanation.

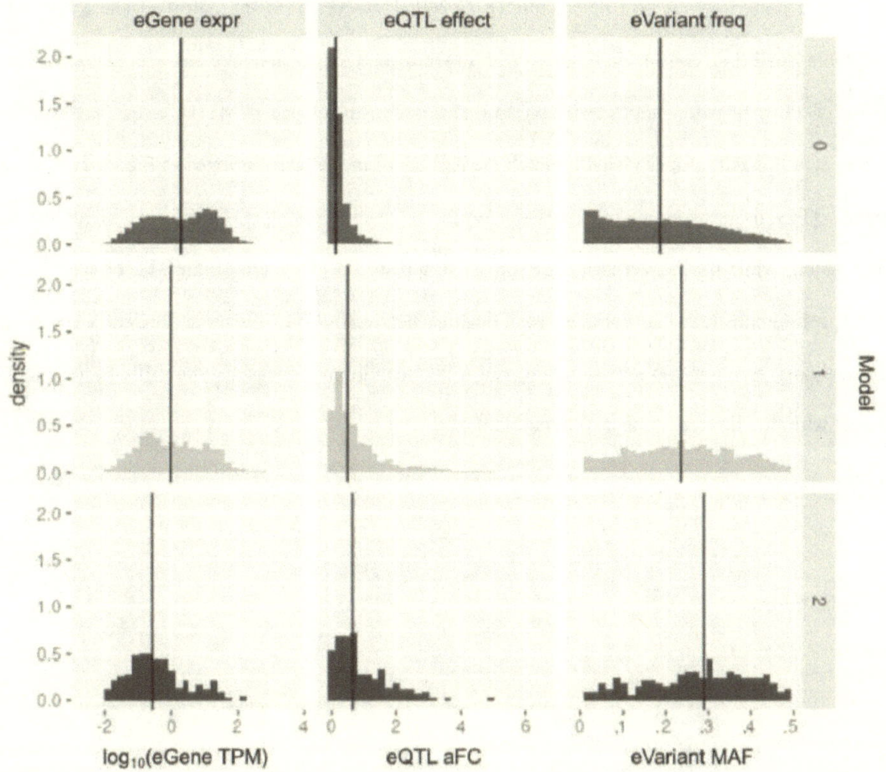

Figure 2.5: eGene, eQTL, and eVariant features of eQTLs by model. Density histograms of various features of top eQTLs are plotted per model (0 = flat, 1 = linear, 2 = bell-curve). Medians are plotted as vertical black lines.

We next visually inspected data from bell curve eQTL examples, including allele specific expression (ASE)-based effect sizes. ASE-based effect sizes averaged across individuals heterozygous for the lead eQTL variant and population-based effect sizes correlate but are not identical, with correlation rhos ranging from 0.75 to 0.84 in GTEx tissues (GTEx Consortium 2020). We visually inspected scatterplots of ASE-based aFC vs. median tissue TPM to see if the bell curve patterns were still reasonable [FIG 2C]. However, ASE-based effect sizes were not available in all tissues, especially those with lower eGene expression. We also calculated within-tissue eQTL-expression slopes based on ASE aFC and log10(eGene TPM). Three eQTL examples where within-tissue slopes visually match the bell curve model are displayed in Figure 2. In these three eQTLs, tissues with lower expression appear to have increasing eQTL effects with increasing expression, while tissues with higher expression appear to have decreasing eQTL effects. These examples demonstrate that complex relationships between eQTL effects and eGene expression exist, though true non-monotonic relationships between the two measures are difficult to reliably detect with this limited number of datapoints.

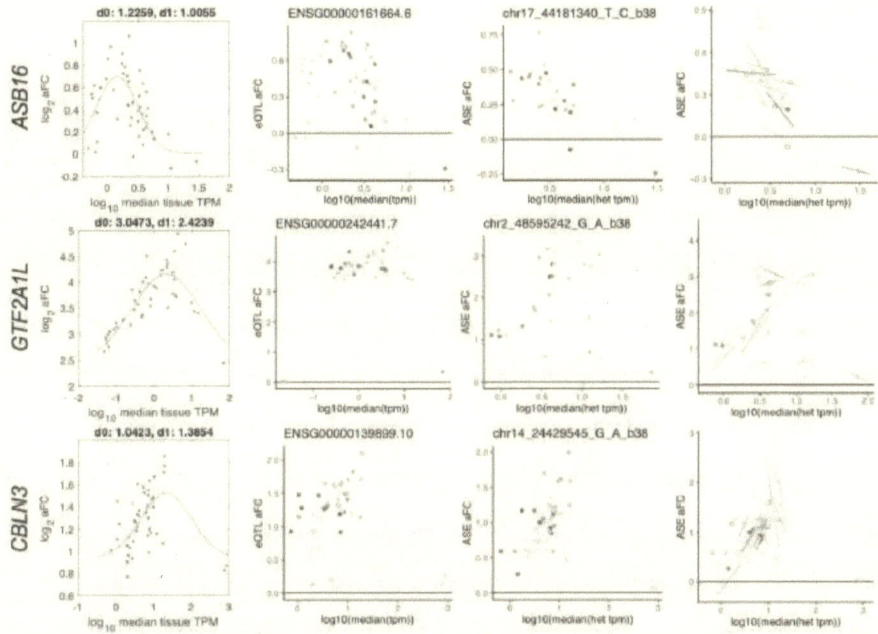

Figure 2.6: Examples of non-monotonic relationships between eGene expression and eQTL effect sizes. Cross-tissue data for eQTLs for three genes (*ASB16*, *GTF2A1L*, *CBLN3*). First column: Quantile-normalized aFC vs. $\log_{10}$(eGene TPM) across tissues, plotted with the best fit M2 model in red. Second column: Non-normalized aFC vs. $\log_{10}$(eGene TPM) across tissues. Third column: Allele-specific-expression-based aFC vs. $\log_{10}$(eGene TPM) in eQTL-variant-heterozygous individuals across tissues. Fourth column: Within-tissue slopes of Allele-specific-expression-based aFC vs. $\log_{10}$(eGene TPM) across eQTL-variant-heterozygous individuals.

2.3.4 Patterns of GWAS genes across tissues

We next investigated cross-tissue gene expression and eQTL patterns of genes associated with GWAS loci to try to gain insight into biological mechanisms of phenotype and disease. We analyzed data from 73 GWASs with previously identified colocalization between GWAS signals and GTEx eQTLs, and we identified 2,157 GWAS-eQTL ENLOC loci, corresponding to 1,110 colocalized genes and 42 GWAS traits. We also looked at the location of these loci and identified

1,096 nearest genes. 697 of the identified loci had different colocalized and nearest genes, and the union of all colocalized and nearest genes is referred to as "GWAS genes."

We next examined eQTL effects and eGene expression for GWAS genes versus all protein-coding and lncRNA genes. For each gene, we determined the discovery tissue of its top eQTL as well as the tissue with the highest gene expression, and we counted how many times each tissue met these criteria per gene set [FIG 2.7]. We saw some interesting patterns emerge for top eQTLs and max gene expression as well as between GWAS genes and all genes. For instance, we observed that testis had the largest number of all genes with the highest expression or as the discovery tissue, but the magnitude of its lead was decreased or eliminated when investigating only GWAS genes. We also saw that blood was often the discovery tissue of top eQTLs for all genes and GWAS genes, while blood and LCLs were often the tissues with the highest gene expression for GWAS genes. Tissues that are often discovery tissues of top eQTL are likely skewed towards tissues with larger sample sizes, as these tissues have a larger number of significant eQTLs. The causes of tissues with frequent high gene expression are more difficult to interpret. However, tissues that have high expression or large eQTL effect sizes for GWAS genes may be more relevant to the disease etiology of the tested GWAS traits. We investigated this hypothesis further by analyzing which tissues showed high gene expression and large eQTL effects sizes for different categories of GWAS traits.

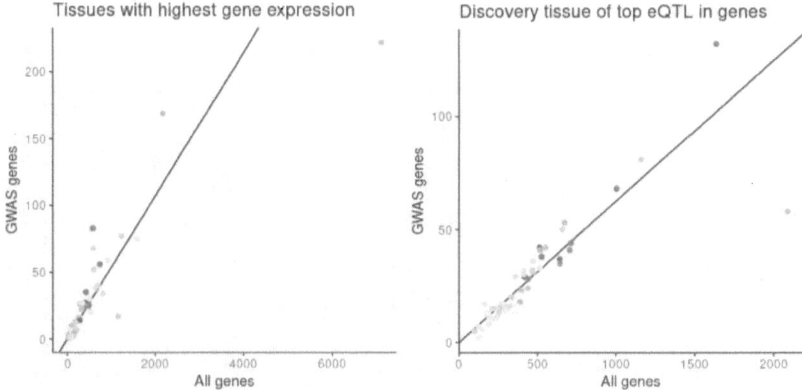

Figure 2.7: Properties of GWAS genes. Left) GTEx tissues plotted by number of GWAS genes with the highest gene expression vs. all genes with the highest gene expression. **Right)** GTEx tissues plotted by number of GWAS genes with the top eQTL vs. all genes with the top eQTL. Black lines plot expected number of GWAS genes based on number of all genes.

For each GWAS trait, we determined which tissue group (blood, brain, immune, or metabolic) may exhibit primary effects that lead to the disease's symptoms, and we analyzed where these tissues ranked in terms of gene expression and eQTL effects for GWAS genes associated with each trait. Since tissues are not evenly distributed across all genes, we compared our GWAS gene statistics to the distribution across all genes [FIG 2.8]. We found that GWAS genes had significantly higher effect sizes and expressions levels in the trait-relevant tissues than expected based on tissue median ranks in the background gene set (Paired Wilcoxon sign test, $p < 10^{-3}$) [TABLE 2.1]. These results suggest that both eQTL effect size and expression level carry relevant information about the tissue that mediates downstream GWAS phenotype effects of genetic variants.

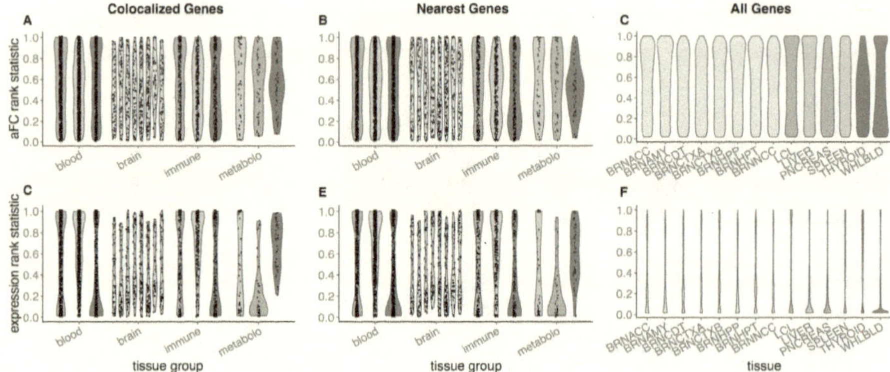

Figure 2.8: Tissue rank statistics of effect size and expression for GWAS and all genes. In GWAS Genes plots (A, B, D, E), each dot represents the rank statistic of a tissue in a GWAS gene. Tissue-gene pairs are plotted for colocalized genes (A, D) and nearest genes (B, E) for aFC (A, B) and expression (D, E) rank statistics. In All Genes plots, aFC (C) and expression (F) rank statistics are plotted for all protein-coding and lncRNA genes, for reference.

Table 2.1: aFC and expression rank statistics of GWAS genes vs. all genes.

Gene selection	Rank method	Tissue-gene pairs	Median rank GWAS	Median rank null	P-value
colocalization	aFC	3492	0.531	0.510	1.52e-04
nearest	aFC	3341	0.542	0.510	3.58e-06
colocalization	expr	3503	0.519	0.222	2.62e-294
nearest	expr	3460	0.481	0.222	4.57e-255

2.4 Discussion

We investigated cross-tissue patterns of eQTL effects and gene expression and discovered complex regulatory patterns that suggest that the relationship between eQTL effects and gene expression is non-trivial. When analyzing the relationship of eQTL effect size and eGene expression across tissues, we found both increasing and decreasing correlations in roughly equal amounts (increasing = 1034, decreasing = 937), totaling to 7.4% of all tested eQTLs. These correlated eQTLs had higher eQTL effect magnitudes and larger minor allele frequencies than non-correlated eQTLs, likely reflective of their wider variability and higher power to detect patterns, and we also observed that positively-correlated eQTLs had lower eGene expression than negatively-correlated eQTLs, which may have biological relevance. We also found 233 eQTLs with non-monotonic relationships between eQTL effect size and eGene expression, highlighting that complex regulatory relationship between eQTLs and eGene expression. Finally, we investigated GWAS trait genes as defined by nearest genes and colocalized eGenes to GWAS loci. We found that GWAS genes had higher gene expression and larger eQTL effects in the putative biologically relevant tissues for the GWAS trait.

One interesting finding was the presence of both positively- and negatively-correlated eQTLs, which confirm previous reports of both positive and negative relationships between eGene expression and eQTL effects under immune stimulation (Kim-Hellmuth et al. 2017; Gutierrez-Arcelus et al. 2020). While both correlation directions had higher eQTL effect magnitudes and larger minor allele frequencies than non-correlated eQTLs, we found that positively-correlated eQTLs had lower eGene expression than negatively-correlated eQTLs. Given the discovery of many non-monotonic relationships between eQTL effects and eGene expression levels, these results are consistent with the idea that many genes may show increasing and then decreasing eQTL effects across the entire gene expression spectrum, but we are only able to observe single correlation directions because the measured eGene expression does not encompass the entire range. The non-monotonic pattern could be explained by eQTL detection and expression saturation: at very low gene expression levels, we would not have power to detect reliably measure the gene, thus we would not have power to observe any eQTL effects. As gene expression increases, we would be able to reliably measure eGene expression and detect eQTL effects. However, at very high gene expression levels, perhaps cells are maximizing transcription from both alleles, thus there is no longer an observable eQTL as both alleles are being maximally expressed. This theory would result in increasing eQTL effects from low to medium eGene expression levels and decreasing eQTL effects from medium to high eGene expression levels and is explored more in *Chapter 3*. However, we likely were underpowered to accurately detect non-monotonic relationships across only 49 tissues, thus this hypothesis remains highly speculatory.

Our exploration of GWAS genes showed higher gene expression and larger eQTL effect sizes in relevant trait tissues, suggesting that examining both may be the best approach for understanding tissues that are causally relevant for human GWAS loci. Interestingly, results for nearest genes and colocalized genes appeared very similar, with both showing significantly higher gene expression and eQTL effect size than all genes in the relevant tissues. This brings up recent research that has suggested that colocalization approaches may be ill-equipped to pinpoint GWAS genes, because true GWAS genes tend to have highly conserved regulation which would impede the presence and discovery of eQTL effects (Wang and Goldstein 2020). However, this theory directly conflicts with our discovery of larger effect sizes for both types of GWAS genes, and further investigation is needed.

Our research highlights the complex gene regulation patterns across tissues. We confirm previously reported bi-directional relationships between gene expression and allelic effects across contexts, showing that eQTL effects cannot be explained by on versus off gene expression across tissues. We find that both gene expression and eQTL effects are higher in GWAS genes in relevant tissues, implying that they both may be informative for determining relevant tissues for traits with unknown etiologies. These analyses highlight the complex relationships between eQTL effects and gene expression across tissues, emphasizing the need for further research into the tissue specificity of regulatory variant effects.

Chapter 3: Transcription factor regulation of genetic variant effects[2]

3.1 Introduction

Gene expression is regulated by local genomic sequence and can be affected by genetic variants. In the human population, tens of thousands of *cis*-regulatory variants have been discovered by expression quantitative trait locus (eQTL) mapping that associates genetic variation to gene expression levels. These variants are enriched to fall in *cis*-regulatory elements and transcription factor binding sites (GTEx Consortium 2015; Gaffney et al. 2012; Kilpinen et al. 2013), implying that many eQTLs act via allelic difference in transcription factor affinity. However, specific mechanisms of individual eQTL effects and their variation across tissues or other contexts remain elusive. Understanding eQTL mechanisms, as well as the contexts in which they are active, can shed light on the regulatory code of the genome and how genetic variation perturbs this regulation.

---

[2] This chapter is adapted from Flynn, E. D., Tsu, A. L., Kasela, S., Kim-Hellmuth, S., Aguet, F., Ardlie, K. G., Bussemaker, H. J., Mohammadi P. & Lappalainen, T. (2021). Transcription factor regulation of eQTL activity across individuals and tissues (p. 2021.07.20.453075). doi:10.1101/2021.07.20.453075

Supplementary Figures and Tables available Supplementary Figures and Tables are available at https://www.biorxiv.org/content/10.1101/2021.07.20.453075v2.supplementary-material.

Genetic, gene expression, eQTL, fine-mapping, and GWAS colocalization data used in these analyses were provided by the GTEx Consortium. Athena Tsu ran the protein-based TF-eQTL correlations, performed enrichment analysis for the ADASTRA allele-specific binding data, and investigated TF-eQTL examples including the IKZF1-*APBB1IP* eQTL interaction. Sarah Kim-Hellmuth provided XCell cell type composition enrichment estimates. All remaining analyses were performed by Elise Flynn.

Multiple efforts have sought to catalog eQTL effects across different contexts. The GTEx Consortium profiled gene expression in 49 tissues across 838 donors and discovered eQTLs for 1,260-18,795 genes per tissue (GTEx Consortium et al. 2017; GTEx Consortium 2020). Approximately a third of these eQTLs were estimated to be active in all or almost all tissues, while a fifth were estimated to be active in five or fewer tissues. Further work using computational cell type deconvolution has discovered approximately three thousand GTEx eQTLs whose effects are likely cell-type-specific (Kim-Hellmuth et al. 2020). Additional context-specific eQTL effects have been assayed in a variety of settings, including during immune stimulation (Alasoo et al. 2018; Kim-Hellmuth et al. 2017), cell stress (Ward et al. 2020; Dombroski et al. 2010), cell differentiation (Strober et al. 2019), and drug or nutrient exposure (Findley et al. 2021; Moyerbrailean et al. 2016; Knowles et al. 2018).

However, few studies have been conducted to investigate what causes eQTL context specificity, i.e., why eQTLs are differentially active across contexts. Some of this variation is of course explained by gene expression: genes that are not expressed will not have a measurable eQTL. However, multiple studies have found that the link between gene expression and eQTL effect is not straightforward, observing both increasing and decreasing allelic effects with increasing gene expression (Gutierrez-Arcelus et al. 2020; GTEx Consortium 2020). When investigating the tissue variability of GTEx eQTLs, we discovered that ~4% of eQTLs show increasing effects with increasing gene expression across tissues, and ~4% show decreasing effects (GTEx Consortium 2020). These findings show that the context variability of eQTL effects cannot be explained by gene expression alone and must depend on other features, such as chromatin accessibility, enhancer looping, or variable levels of transcription factor binding.

Determining eQTLs' mechanisms of action is challenging. The first obstacle lies in identifying the causal variant(s) of a locus from the typically numerous associated variants in high linkage disequilibrium (LD). Putatively functional variants can be pinpointed by statistical fine-mapping approaches, complemented with genomic annotations such as regions of open chromatin, TF binding sites predicted by motifs, or allele-specific binding of TF ChIP-seq data (Kichaev et al. 2014, 2019; GTEx Consortium 2020; Weissbrod et al. 2020; Kubota and Suyama 2021). However, these annotations suffer from both low specificity and low sensitivity. In terms of specificity, a large percentage of variants in the genome overlap some functional annotation; for instance, Gaffney et al found that 40% of SNPs in eQTLs overlapped a DNAse I hypersensitive site or histone-modified region (Gaffney et al. 2012). In terms of sensitivity, functional data may be missing for the context in which the eQTL is active, and especially the highly informative allelic binding data are relatively sparse (J. Chen et al. 2016; Tehranchi et al. 2016; Abramov et al. 2021). While experimental assays that directly measure regulatory effects of variants are increasing in scale, they may miss *in vivo* interactions or chromatin-specific regulation (Inoue et al. 2017), and intensive experimental approaches to directly profile the effects and mechanisms of genetic variants in an eQTL (Lou et al. 2009; Meyer et al. 2013; Gupta et al. 2017; Zhao et al. 2020) are difficult to conduct in a high-throughput manner.

One thing made clear by functional annotation data is that both eQTLs and chromatin-QTLs are enriched in known TF binding sites (GTEx Consortium et al. 2017; Gaffney et al. 2012; Waszak et al. 2015). Given that TFs are one of the few sequence-specific interactors with the genome, it follows that noncoding eQTLs may exert their effects by altering TF binding, which would then affect chromatin accessibility, histone modifications, and gene expression. Adding to the hypothesis that TF binding may control eQTL variability, many cross-tissue eQTLs are enriched in TF binding sites for TFs with broad activity, while tissue-specific eQTLs are enriched for those relevant to their observed tissue (Y. He et al. 2020). By determining which TF's binding is being altered by an eQTL, we would be able to identify its mechanism of action, as well as understand what could be regulating the eQTL's context variability.

In this study, we set out to discover TF regulators of eQTLs by identifying eQTL effects that correlate with TF levels across or within tissues, using primarily GTEx data. We use the natural variation of TF levels between tissues, individuals, and conditions to elucidate mechanisms of action of eQTL regulatory variants and understand the context specificity of eQTL effects. We hypothesize that a portion of the observed context variability of an eQTL may be explained by the level of the TFs that bind to the eQTL to regulate gene expression [Fig. 3.1A-C]. In the simplest form of the model, an allele may increase the affinity of an activating TF in a *cis*-regulatory site, which would lead to higher gene expression of that allele [Fig. 3.1A]. However, at low TF levels, the TF would not bind to either allele, resulting in the same low level of background gene expression from each allele. Conversely, at very high TF levels of saturated binding, even the lower affinity allele could bind the TF, and both alleles would have equal gene expression. This would translate to increasing and then decreasing eQTL effects as TF levels increase [Fig. 3.1C]. Other models are explored in the supplement [SFig. 1].

Our approach links variation in TF levels to variation in eQTL effect size and requires no additional datatypes to be captured, using the same genetic and gene expression data that are used for eQTL discovery. It offers a novel approach to understanding regulatory variant context specificity that can refine and complement existing approaches based on statistical fine-mapping and functional genomic experiments. Applying it to GTEx data, we find thousands of interactions between TF levels and eQTL effects both across tissues and within tissues which represent potential TF regulators of eQTL effects, and we validate these data using numerous approaches and datasets. Finally, we highlight an example of an IKZF1-regulated eQTL that colocalizes with multiple GWAS blood traits, evidencing how this TF-based model can be used to unravel effects on human health and disease.

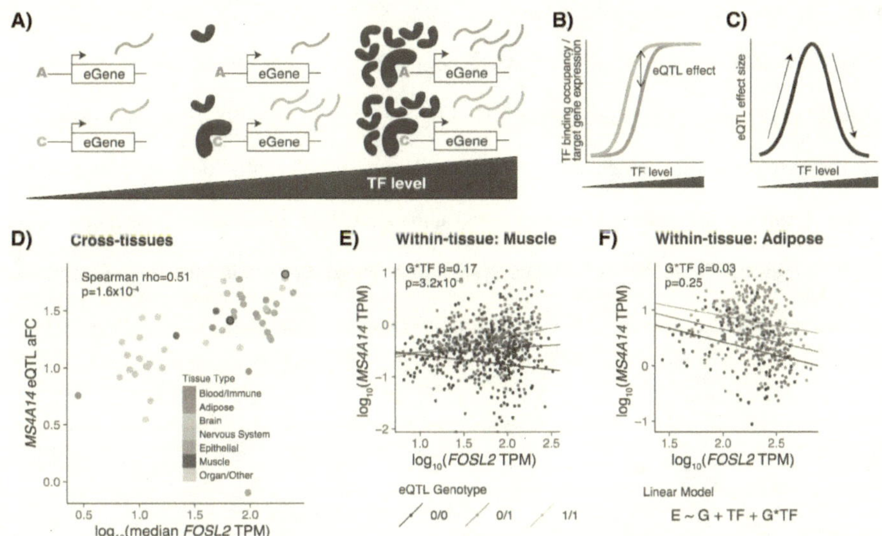

Figure 3.1: TF model of eQTL effects. A) TF binding to an eQTL variant with different allelic TF affinities is depicted at low, medium, and high TF levels. **B)** TF binding occupancy, resulting in target gene expression, for the two eQTL alleles across TF levels. **C)** Difference in expression of alleles or eQTL effect size, quantified as $\log_2$ allelic fold change, across TF levels. Our applied models only examine monotonic effects, which can be imagined as different sides of the hill. **D)** Tissues are plotted by eQTL effect size vs. median TF expression for an example *MS4A14* eQTL and the FOSL2 TF. Cross-tissue TF-eQTL interactions are discovered by a Spearman correlation of these two measures, or with TF protein levels for the protein-based analysis. **E) & F)** Individuals are plotted by eGene expression vs. TF expression in Skeletal Muscle (E) or Adipose Visceral (F) tissue and are shaded by the genotype of the eQTL variant. Within-tissue TF-eQTL interactions are discovered using a linear regression interaction model of normalized eGene expression by TF level, genotype, and TF level by genotype. Linear regression lines are plotted or each genotype. In Muscle, a TF-eQTL interaction is present, as the difference gets larger as TF expression increases. In Adipose, an eQTL is present, but no TF-eQTL interaction is observed.

3.2 Materials and Methods

3.2.1 GTEx data

For the bulk of our analysis, we used the GTEx v8 dataset, including whole genome sequencing for 838 individuals and mRNA sequencing from 15,201 samples across 49 tissues [Table 3.1, STable 1]. RNA-seq data were aligned using STAR v2.5.3a, and gene counts were based on GENCODE Release 26 and analyzed using RNA-SeQC (GTEx Consortium 2020). *cis*-eQTL calculations in each tissue and Caviar fine-mapping 95% confidence sets for those eQTLs were also previously generated [Table 3.1] (GTEx Consortium 2020). High-throughput mass spectrometry protein measurements were separately available for 201 GTEx samples across 32 tissues (Jiang et al. 2020) [Table 3.1, STable 1]. GTEx tissues were categorized into Blood/Immune, Adipose, Brain, Nervous System (non-brain), Epithelial, Muscle, or Organ/Other via a cursory literature search on biological composition and function.

Table 3.1: Data Sources.

Data Type	Publication DOI / Citation	Website
GTEx v8 genetic, gene expression, eQTL, and fine-mapping data	10.1126/science.aaz1776 / (GTEx Consortium 2020)	https://gtexportal.org/home/
GTEx protein data	10.1016/j.cell.2020.08.036 / (Jiang et al. 2020)	
GTEx GWAS colocalization	10.1186/s13059-020-02252-4 / (Barbeira et al. 2021)	
ENCODE TF ChIP-seq peaks	Multiple experiments	https://www.encodeproject.org/search/?type=Experiment
HOCOMOCO TF motifs	10.1093/nar/gkx1106 / (Kulakovskiy et al. 2018)	https://hocomoco11.autosome.ru/
ADASTRA allele-specific binding data	10.1038/s41467-021-23007-0 / (Abramov et al. 2021)	https://adastra.autosome.ru/susan
HEK293-TLR4 IRF1 knockdown experiment	10.1101/2020.02.21.959734 / (Brandt, Kim-Hellmuth, et al. 2020)	
HEK293-TLR4 genome sequence	10.1038/ncomms5767 / (Lin et al. 2014)	http://hek293genome.org/v2
Gene-by-environment interactions	10.7554/eLife.67077 / (Findley et al. 2021)	

3.2.2 Filtering variants

We limit our analysis to variants where we have prior evidence to suggest that this could be a variant affecting gene expression that is regulated by a TF. We filtered for variants that matched four criteria: 1) >=5% minor allele frequency in GTEx v8 samples; 2) present in a Caviar fine-mapped 95% credible set for an eQTL in any GTEx tissue; 3) overlap an ENCODE TF ChIP-seq peak for at least one of 169 TFs; 4) match a HOCOMOCO consensus sequence motif for at least one of 169 TFs. We used ENCODE narrowPeak regions in all available experiments that passed filtering criteria (as of January 2020) and HOCOMOCO v11 IUPAC consensus motifs [Table 2]. For the ENCODE TF ChIP-seq overlap, we used ChIP-seq optimal irreproducible discovery rate (IDR) threshold peak files for experiments with a biological replicate, no red or orange audit categories, and no experimental conditions. We used a union of regions if multiple IDR files were available per TF. For HOCOMOCO TF motif matching, we converted the IUPAC consensus sequence motif to a regular-expression string for both the forward and reverse-compliment motif, trimming any less confident bases (lowercase letters) from the ends of the sequence. We extracted the genomic sequence surrounding each variant (motif length minus one on either side of the variant) using samtools, and we used grep to check if the forward or reverse-compliment motif was present in the reference and/or the alternative alleles. The above filtering left us with 473,057 variants. Using the Caviar fine-mapping data, we associated each filtered variant with one or more eGenes, which resulted in 1,032,124 eVariant-eGene pairs across 32,151 genes.

3.2.3 Within-tissue TF-eQTL interactions

For our within-tissue TF-eQTL interaction discovery, we selected twenty tissues that best represented all 49 GTEx eQTL tissues based on gene expression clustering. We clustered tissues based on median TPM across all genes using Euclidean distances and Ward.D clustering, cut the resulting tree to generate twenty clusters, and selected the tissue with the largest sample size from each cluster. If a tissue was removed for cell type composition variability (below), the next largest tissue was selected from the cluster, if one was available.

For each selected tissue, we applied an eQTL interaction model to discover TF-eQTL interactions on gene expression. We ran tensorQTL software per TF and per tissue for 32,151 genes and all filtered variants within a 10 mega-base window of the transcription start site, inputting individuals' genotypes, normalized eGene expression, and normalized TF expression for each eQTL-TF pair, as well as genotype principal components and tissue covariates described in The GTEx Consortium, 2020 (GTEx Consortium 2020). TensorQTL software applied a gene-level p-value correction based on the effective number of independent variants tested per gene, estimated with eigenMT (emt), and selected the variant with the lowest p-value per gene (Taylor-Weiner et al. 2019; Davis et al. 2016). We then applied a Benjamini-Hochberg (BH) correction to the emt-corrected p-values across each tissue and TF. For all TF-eQTL interactions with BH FDR <= 20%, we selected those where the top TF-eQTL variant had a significant eQTL signal in the respective tissue and where the gene was not the implicated TF.

We removed four tissues with high cell type composition variability so that our results were not dominated by non-causal TF-eQTL relationships due to cell type composition (Whole Blood, Fibroblast, Colon, Stomach), and we removed one tissue due to its high number of results and unique gene expression patterns (Testis). Cell type composition was estimated in Kim-Hellmuth et al., 2020 (Kim-Hellmuth et al. 2020): briefly, XCell was used to calculate enrichment of cell-type-specific gene expression signals in GTEx samples (Aran, Hu, and Butte 2017). Since these estimates were not all experimentally validated, we ignored cell type estimates with high variability across tissues (aDC, iDC) [SFig. 5]. Four cell type estimates had high variability in a GTEx tissue (variance > 0.04; Th2 cells in fibroblasts, epithelial cells in the colon, epithelial cells in the stomach, and basophils in blood) and those tissues were removed from the analysis to avoid strong cell type interaction signals in our results. Stomach clustered with other tissues [SFig. 4], so we added the next largest tissue in that group, Pancreas, to our within-tissue TF-eQTL analysis.

3.2.4 Cross-tissue TF-eQTL correlations

We correlated eQTL effect sizes and TF expression levels across up to 49 GTEx tissues. We used the aFC software package to calculate eQTL effect sizes based on log2 allelic fold change (aFC) for all eVariant-eGene pairs in each tissue (Mohammadi et al. 2017b), using genotype principal components and tissue covariates described in The GTEx Consortium, 2020 (GTEx Consortium 2020). We determined the median TF level per tissue based on transcripts per million (TPM). Then we performed a cross-tissue Spearman correlation of eQTL aFC and TF median TPM for each eQTL-TF pair in all tissues with median eGene expression greater than 0 TPM, i.e., in all tissues where the eQTL target gene was sufficiently expressed. We tested 1-249 eVariants per eGene, and we selected the top variant per gene and calculated a corrected p-value using the effective number of independent variants tested per gene. We defined the effective number of tests per gene as the number of eigenvectors needed to capture 95% of the variance in the GTEx genotype matrix of all tested variants, using the Gao method in the poolr package (Gao, Starmer, and Martin 2008). We then performed a Benjamini-Hochberg TF-level correction of the meff-corrected p-values across the top variants of each gene, and we selected variants with up to a 5% false discovery rate (FDR).

For our protein-based analysis, we used a similar approach, substituting TF protein levels for TF expression levels. We examined median protein levels in 32 GTEx tissues using normalized high-throughput mass spectrometry data (Jiang et al. 2020). We filtered for TFs with at least 20 unique protein values across tissues, then performed a cross-tissue Spearman correlation of eQTL aFC and TF median protein level. We tested 1,032,124 eQTLs and 72 TFs using the same p-value calculation procedure described above, then selected variants with up to a 20% FDR.

3.2.5 Dataset comparison

We tested for TF-eQTL sharing across multiple datasets: cross-tissue expression-based, cross-tissue protein-based, and each within-tissue expression-based dataset. We performed Fisher's tests based on every TF-eGene pair's presence in the significant interactions from each dataset. For comparisons with cross-tissue protein-based data, we only used TF-eGene pairs for 72 TFs tested in the protein data.

3.2.6 TF binding overlap enrichment

We tested whether our predicted TF-eQTL interactions overlap TF binding sites (TFBS) based on two orthogonal datasets: ENCODE TF ChIP-seq peaks and HOCOMOCO predicted TF binding motifs [Table 2]. Given the complicated structure of our data, with multiple variants tested per gene and LD between variants, we used an expectation/observation model to test TFBS overlap enrichment of TF-eQTL interactions.

For each TF (f), we calculated the number of expected overlaps per gene (g) based on the number of variants tested (v) and the probability that any variant overlapped that annotation (p), and compared that to the observed number variants that overlap the annotation (o):

$$S_{f,g} = obs_{f,g} - exp_{f,g} = o_{f,g} - v_g * p_f \qquad \text{(Eq 3.1)}$$

We then averaged the per gene statistics across all genes with a significant TF-eQTL interaction (G_f):

$$S_f = \frac{\sum_{g \in G_f} S_{f,g}}{|G_f|} \qquad \text{(Eq 3.2)}$$

And we averaged across all 169 TFs to get our final enrichment statistic:

$$S_{overlap} = \frac{\sum_{f=1}^{169} S_f * |G_f|}{\sum_{f=1}^{169} |G_f|} \quad \text{(Eq 3.3)}$$

The resulting statistic can be interpreted as the average extra number of overlaps per gene. For instance, an overlap enrichment statistic of 0.01 would mean that we observed 0.01 more variants with overlap per TF-eQTL gene than expected – or one additional overlap per 100 genes.

Permutations were carried out by shuffling overlap annotations across all tested variants and recalculating the overlap statistic 10^4 times. Permutation p-values were calculated by counting the number of times the permuted TF statistic is larger or smaller than the observed statistic, adding one, dividing by the number of permutations, and multiplying by two for a two-sided test.

3.2.7 Allele-specific TF binding validation

We examined TF allele-specific binding (ASB) data to determine if our high-confidence set of potential TF regulators led to altered TF binding *ex vivo*. We based our analysis on the ADASTRA dataset (Susan version), which contains a meta-analysis of allele-specific TF binding results from over 7,000 TF ChIP-seq experiments [Table 4.1] (Abramov et al. 2021). Similar to our TFBS overlap enrichment analysis, we used an expectation/observation model to test allele-specific binding of TF-eQTL interactions, then permuted allele-specific binding annotations to calculate the enrichment significance.

For the un-matched TF ASB overlap analysis, we calculated the number of expected variants with ASB per gene based on the number of tested variants that were assayed in the ASB dataset (v) and the probability that any variant had ASB for any TF (p). We then compared the expected to the observed number of variants with ASB (o) in each gene, and we averaged across all genes that had a significant TF-eQTL interaction for any TF (G_{any}):

$$S_{any} = \frac{\sum_{g \in G_{any}} S_{,g}}{|G_{any}|} \qquad \text{(Eq 3.4)}$$

For our matched TF analysis, we calculated the number of expected variants with ASB per gene based on the number of tested variants that were assayed in the ASB dataset (v) and the probability that any variant had ASB for the specified TF (p). We then compared the expected to the observed number of variants with ASB (o) using the equation for S_g described previously (Eq 1), then averaged the per gene statistics across all correlated genes using the equation for S_f (Eq 2).

The overall enrichment was calculated using S_g and S_f, with genes with a significant TF-eQTL interaction per TF (G_f) and 124 total TFs, using the full equation:

$$S_{matched} = \frac{\sum_{f=1}^{124} \sum_{g \in G_f} o_{f,g} - v_g * p_f}{\sum_{f=1}^{124} |G_f|} \qquad \text{(Eq 3.5)}$$

We then permuted ASB annotations across all tested variants and recalculated the ASB statistic 10^4 times. We calculated permutation p-values using the same two-sided test procedure described in our TFBS overlap enrichment analysis.

3.2.8 IRF1 knockdown analysis

Our high confidence set of potential TF regulators included 58 eQTL effects predicted to be regulated by IRF1. To test these, we used a CRISPR-i knockdown of IRF1 in TLR4-expressing HEK cells (HEK293T) and measured allele-specific expression (ASE) at varying IRF1 levels

[Table 4.1] (Brandt, Kim-Hellmuth, et al. 2020). If we observe that ASE changes with IRF1 levels, this would suggest that IRF1 is truly regulating the effect of the eQTL on gene expression. First, we filtered the aligned HEK293T RNA-seq data for coding variants that had adequate coverage to call ASE: at least 60 reads across all conditions, at least 5% reference allele and 5% alternative allele, and less than 5% of other alleles. Then, we used Fisher's test to compare the allelic balance across all promoter knockdown samples and all control samples. As our test was likely underpowered, we looked at genes with a 0.05 nominal p-value cutoff. We then checked which IRF1-eQTL top variants were heterozygous in the HEK293T cell line using VCF files from Complete Genomics [Table 4.1] (Lin et al. 2014). All seven testable IRF1-eQTL were heterozygous for a top IRF1-eQTL variant in the HEK293T cell line.

3.2.9 Comparison with GxE genes

Gene-by-environment interaction analysis results were attained from Supplemental Table 4 in Findley et al., 2021 [Table 4.1] (Findley et al. 2021). We matched these results by ENSG number with our dual-evidence TF-eQTL genes and used Fisher's exact test to calculate overlap compared to all tested genes in our dataset.

3.2.10 GWAS colocalization

To discover TF regulators of GWAS loci, we examined colocalization of GTEx eQTLs and 76 GWAS traits. We obtained ENLOC colocalization results (regional conditional probability > 0.5) from the GTEx Consortium [Table 4.1] (Wen, Pique-Regi, and Luca 2017; Barbeira et al. 2021) and overlapped these eQTL genes with our high confidence TF-eQTL genes. To test if our TF-eQTLs were enriched to colocalize with GWAS signals, we looked at all significant eQTL genes in any tissue and performed a Fisher's exact test for whether or not the gene had an eQTL that colocalized with a GWAS phenotype and whether or not we found a TF-eQTL interaction for that gene. We also performed a tissue-specific analysis where we looked at all significant eQTL genes in the 16 tissues where we performed within-tissue TF-eQTL discovery, and we performed a Fisher's exact test for whether or not the tissue's eQTL signal colocalized with a GWAS phenotype and whether or not a high confidence TF-eQTL was found for that gene in the tissue. Our list of 205 colocalizing GWAS-eQTLs with a TF-eQTL were based on this tissue-specific comparison and were additionally filtered such that the r^2 of the top TF-eQTL variant and the lead ENLOC colocalizing variant was great than 0.4.

3.3 Results

3.3.1 Selection of putative regulatory variants

For the bulk of our analysis, we used the GTEx v8 dataset, including whole genome sequencing for 838 individuals and RNA sequencing from 73-706 samples across 49 tissues [STable 1]. We focused our analysis on common variants (>5% MAF) that have prior evidence of affecting gene expression and being regulated by a TF [Table 3.2]. We used Caviar fine-mapping of GTEx eQTLs in 49 tissues to select variants that fell into a 95% credible set in at least one tissue (Hormozdiari et al. 2014; GTEx Consortium 2020). We also required evidence that a TF binds in the vicinity of the variant. We focused our analysis on 169 TFs with both ENCODE ChIP-seq and HOCOMOCO motif information and included variants that overlapped at least one ChIP-seq peak and matched at least one motif for these TFs.

Filtering based on an intersection of these fine-mapping and functional annotations left us with 473,057 variants that corresponded to 1,032,124 eQTLs across 32,151 genes. Each variant was associated with a median of two genes, and each gene was associated with a median of 28 variants across tissues [SFig. 2]. Next, we used cross-individual and cross-tissue analyses to discover which of this large number of candidate variants had additional evidence of TF mechanisms underlying their eQTL effects.

Table 3.2: GTEx variant annotations. Overlap of variants with >5% minor allele frequency (MAF) in the GTEx dataset that overlap various eQTL and TF annotations. Percent is based on all 5% MAF variants. Filtering eQTL variants for TF binding sites based on TF ChIP-seq peak overlaps and TF motif matches still results in a large number of potentially causal eQTL variants.

Dataset	>5% MAF GTEx variants	
	Count	Percent
All	6,539,590	-
Caviar fine-mapped set	2,867,556	44%
ENCODE TF ChIP-seq peak	1,425,613	22%
HOCOMOCO TF motif	3,716,312	57%
Intersection	473,057	7%

3.3.2 Interaction of eQTL effects and TF expression levels within tissues

We first investigated how inter-individual variation in TF levels within a tissue impacts eQTL effect size, with the hypothesis that such effects could represent TF regulators of specific eQTLs. We chose 20 diverse tissues that best represented all 49 GTEx eQTL tissues based on gene expression clustering [SFig. 3]. For each of those tissues and each of our 169 TFs, we applied a linear regression with an interaction term to discover TF level - genotype interactions on gene expression for our filtered variants across 32,151 genes, selecting the top eQTL variant per gene for each analysis (Taylor-Weiner et al. 2019) [Fig. 3.1E,F]. We discovered 13 to 39,693 TF-eQTLs (eQTLs with TF interaction) per tissue at a 20% TF-level Benjamini-Hochberg (BH) FDR, with 133,111 relationships supported by at least one tissue [SFig. 4]. These TF-eQTL pairs represent potential TF regulators of eQTL effects.

We observed that five tissues (Whole Blood, Fibroblast, Colon, Stomach, and Testis) were outliers in the number of TF-eQTLs, which could not be explained by tissue sample size alone [SFig. 4]. Analysis of *in silico* cell type estimates revealed that four of these tissues (Whole Blood, Fibroblast, Colon, and Stomach) had particularly high inter-individual variability in cell type composition [SFig. 5]. Assuming that this high cell type composition variability was likely contributing to the large number of TF-eQTLs, we removed these tissues from our analysis so that our TF-eQTL results were not dominated by non-causal correlations of TFs with cell type composition. We also removed the Testis tissue due to its outlier status in previously reported gene expression and *trans*-regulation analyses (GTEx Consortium 2015; GTEx Consortium et al. 2017), so that TF-eQTLs in this one tissue would not dominate the results.

Our final within-tissue dataset consisted of 26,038 TF-eQTL relationships supported by at least one tissue, of which 2,315 were supported by multiple tissues [Fig. 3.2A; SFig. 6]. Some TFs with many interacting eQTLs in a tissue made clear biological sense. For instance, the TFs with the most interactions in Brain Cortex and Nucleus Accumbens tissues were BCL11A and MEF2D, respectively, both of which are involved in neuronal functions (Simon, Wiegreffe, and Britsch 2020; Akhtar et al. 2012), and the TF with the most interactions in Adipose tissue was CEBPA, which is a key driver of adipogenesis (Gregoire, Smas, and Sul 1998) [Fig. 3.2A]. We see that 90/120 tissue pairs were enriched for one another's TF-eQTLs (OR = 14.1 to 2251, Fisher's exact test, all $p < 0.05$) [Fig. 3.2C]. All those pairs with a negative direction of enrichment included a brain tissue and/or the lymphoblastoid cell line and did not have any overlapping TF-eQTL interactions, likely due to the small sample sizes and these tissue types being highly distinct from others (all ORs = 0, Fisher's exact test ps = 1) (GTEx Consortium 2020). In general, within-tissue TF-eQTL relationships follow a similar clustering pattern to tissue gene expression [SFig. 3]. These results highlight unique and shared potential TF regulators of eQTL effects within different tissue contexts.

3.3.3 Correlation of eQTL effect sizes and TF levels across tissues

To obtain further insights into TFs driving eQTL effect size variation between tissues, we next investigated how TF levels across the 49 GTEx tissues correlated with eQTL effect sizes. We calculated log2 allelic fold change effect sizes (aFCs) in every GTEx tissue for each filtered variant-gene pair; by ignoring eQTL significance cutoffs, we captured tissues lacking eQTL effects and avoided power differences in eQTL detection caused by varying tissue sample sizes. We correlated aFCs for each eQTL with expression levels for each of 169 TFs [Fig. 3.1D] and selected the top eQTL variant per gene for each TF. We found 420,248 TF-eQTL correlations at a 5% TF-level BH FDR [Fig. 3.2B]. These TF-eQTL pairs represent potential TF regulators of eQTL effects that may explain the variability of these eQTLs across tissues. Many of the TFs with the most correlations in the cross-tissue analysis were involved in immune (ELF1, IRF2, RELB, STAT3, RELA) or hormone response (THRA) (Seifert et al. 2019; Taniguchi et al. 2001; Hayden and Ghosh 2011; Hillmer et al. 2016; Ortiga-Carvalho, Sidhaye, and Wondisford 2014) [Fig. 3.2B]. Though we discovered many more potential TF-eQTL relationships across tissues than within tissues, the two sets of TF-eQTL interactions are enriched for one another (OR = 2.43, Fisher's exact test $p < 10^{-300}$), and cross-tissue correlations showed a positive direction of enrichment for all individual tissues except brain cerebellum [Fig. 3.2C].

Gene expression levels do not always directly correspond to protein levels (Greenbaum et al. 2003; Gry et al. 2009), so we performed a similar correlation analysis using TF protein levels across tissues, as assessed by high-throughput mass spectrometry (Jiang et al. 2020). Protein quantification was available for 72/169 TFs in 20 or more tissues, with one to 11 samples per tissue [STable 1]. We discovered 12,289 TF protein-eQTL correlations at a 20% TF-level BH FDR [Fig. 3.2B]. These protein-based TF-eQTL correlations were not enriched for expression-based cross-tissue or within-tissue TF-eQTL correlations (OR = 0.95, 0.47; Fisher's exact test p = 0.097, 7.9×10^{-7}, respectively) [Fig. 3.2C, SFig. 7]. As discussed in Jiang et al., gene and protein levels may differ due to biological phenomena of RNA dynamics and translational regulation as well as technical variation in mass spectrometry technology that plagues especially lowly expressed proteins (Jiang et al. 2020). Given that TF protein levels are lower than other genes (Wilcoxon rank sum test $p < 10^{-300}$) [SFig. 8] and the number of assayed tissues and samples is small, these protein measurements may be less suitable measurements of TF levels for the purposes of this analysis.

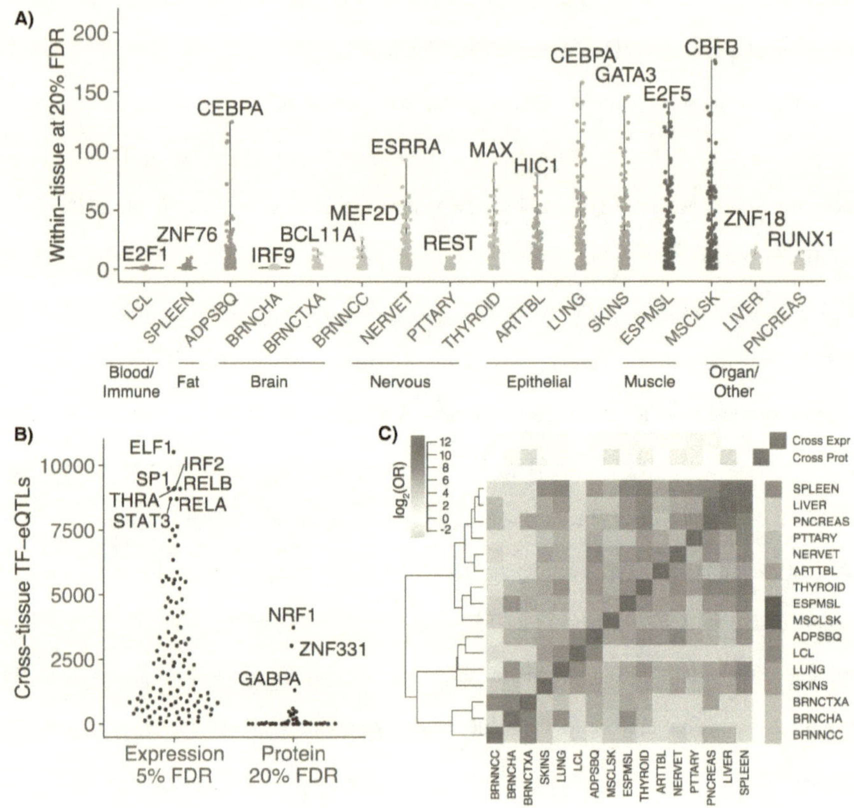

Figure 3.2: Discovered TF-eQTL interactions. A) Number of within-tissue TF-eQTL interactions at 20% FDR is plotted per TF for each tissue analyzed. The TF with the most interactions per tissue is highlighted. **B)** Number of discovered cross-tissue TF-eQTL interactions per TF for expression-based interactions (at 5% FDR) and for protein-based interactions (at 20% FDR). TFs with the most correlations per analysis are highlighted. **C)** Sharing of TF-eQTL interactions between tissues and within/cross-tissues. Red indicates positive enrichment and blue, negative enrichment. Grey squares indicate no shared TF-eQTL gene pairs between the two datasets.

3.3.4 Annotation and TF-binding of TF-eQTL interactions

Next, we set out to evaluate our discovered sets of putative TF regulators of eQTLs, based on orthogonal data of functional annotations and TF binding. We examined four TF-eQTL datasets: cross-tissue expression-based, cross-tissue protein-based, within-tissue expression-based, and at least two lines of expression-based evidence (at least two tissues, or cross-tissue + at least one tissue). First, we examined genomic annotations of the top TF-eQTL variant for each gene and found that all three expression-based datasets were enriched to overlap promoters, 5' UTR, and 3' UTRs compared to all tested eQTL variants [SFig. 9]. This is consistent with overall eQTL enrichments (GTEx Consortium et al. 2017; GTEx Consortium 2015), suggesting that TF-eQTL variants are further enriched for true causal regulatory variants.

We tested whether our four sets of putative TF-eQTL interactions overlapped TF binding sites (TFBS) based on two datasets: ENCODE TF ChIP-seq peaks and HOCOMOCO predicted TF binding motifs. The top TF-eQTL variants showed enrichment for TF ChIP-seq overlap in most datasets and mixed results on TF motif matching enrichment [SFig. 10]. Given the complicated structure of our data, with multiple variants tested per gene and LD between variants [SFig. 2, 11], we set up a more sophisticated test of TFBS overlap enrichment of TF-eQTL interactions to account for this unusual data structure. We compared the observed overlap per gene to a null expectation and calculated significance using a permutation scheme of TFBS overlap annotations (see *Methods*). Our enrichment statistic can be interpreted as the average number of extra variants with overlap per TF-eQTL gene. Both cross-tissue and within-tissue expression-based datasets were significantly enriched for ChIP-seq overlap (cross-tissue enrichment statistic = 0.024, $p < 2 \times 10^{-4}$; within-tissue enrichment statistic = 0.053, $p = 8 \times 10^{-4}$), and cross-tissue expression-based TF-eQTLs showed a small trend of motif matching enrichment (enrichment statistic = 0.004, p =

0.06) [Fig. 3.3A; SFig. 11]. TF-eQTLs with at least two lines of expression-based evidence did not reach nominal significance for ChIP-seq overlap or motif matching, but they showed a similar magnitude of enrichment to the individual datasets [Fig. 3.3A; SFig. 11]. The cross-tissue protein-based TF-eQTL interactions had low enrichment for ChIP-seq overlap and motif matching [Fig. 3.3A; SFig. 10, 11]; thus, taken together with their low concordance with expression-based interactions [Fig. 3.2C], we decided not to pursue these interactions any farther.

Though our discovered expression-based TF-eQTL relationships were generated using only genetic and gene expression data, those eQTLs were more likely to overlap a TFBS of their interacting TF than expected [Fig. 3.3A]. We included all TF-eQTL interactions with at least two lines of expression-based evidence to represent a high-confidence set of putative TF regulators of genetic variant effects. These TF-eQTL genes were also enriched to fall into the regulon of the interacting TF (any regulon set OR = 1.54, Fisher's exact test $p = 1x10^{-17}$) (Garcia-Alonso et al. 2019), with the strongest enrichment seen for regulons defined by co-expression analysis (OR = 2.08, Fisher's exact test $p = 1x10^{-22}$) [Fig. 3.3B]. These 6,262 dual-evidence TF-eQTL interactions, observed across 154 TFs and 1,598 genes, represent potential TF regulators of genetic variant effects [STable 2] that we then analyzed further.

3.3.5 Allele-specific TF binding of dual-evidence TF-eQTL interactions

We next examined TF ChIP-seq allele-specific binding data to determine if our dual-evidence TF regulators of genetic variant effects manifested altered TF binding *ex vivo*. To accomplish this, we used the ADASTRA dataset, which contains allele-specific TF binding (ASB) results from over seven thousand TF ChIP-seq experiments, normalized for cell-type-specific background allelic dosage (Abramov et al. 2021). Like our TFBS overlap enrichment analysis, we compared the observed allele-specific TF binding of TF-eQTL interactions to a null expectation, followed by permutation of ASB annotations to estimate the enrichment significance.

We observed that TF-eQTL variants were significantly more likely to have ASB in general, with any TF (enrichment statistic = 0.09, p=0.002) [Fig. 3.3C]. Testing for the enrichment of ASB for the matching TF-eQTL TF was limited by the sparsity of the ASB data: only 9 out of 124 analyzed TFs were expected to have more than one interacting TF-eQTL with an ASB event [SFig. 13]. However, 8/9 of these TFs showed more ASB than expected, though none to a significant degree [Fig. 3.3C], and the overall enrichment was modest but again non-significant (enrichment statistic = 0.011, p=0.10). These results demonstrate that our dual-evidence TF-eQTL interactions are enriched for variants that alter TF binding, though these data are too sparse to validate this specifically for the implicated TF.

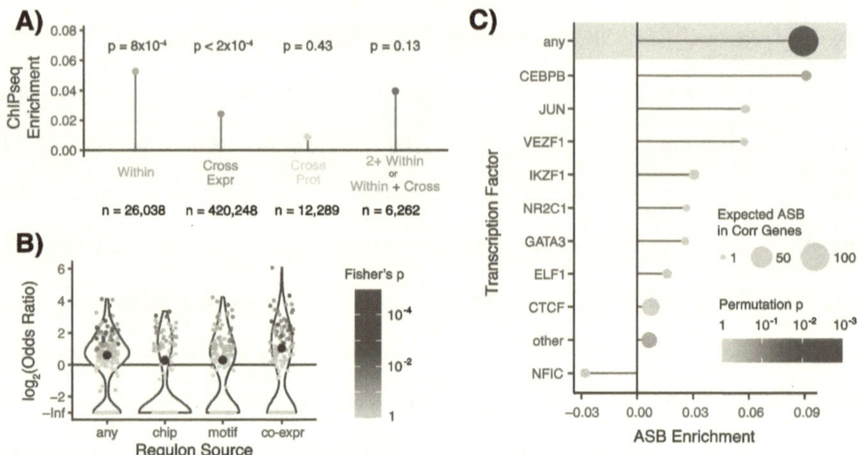

Figure 3.3: TF binding of TF-eQTL interactions. A) Overlap enrichment of TFBS, based on TF ChIP-seq peaks, of TF-eQTL interactions by dataset. Permutation-based p-values are plotted above each measurement. Datasets include within-tissue (blue) interactions, cross-tissue expression-based (red), cross-tissue protein-based (yellow), and TF-eQTL interactions with at least two lines of evidence from cross-tissue expression-based and within-tissue interactions (purple). **B)** The enrichment of target genes with two lines of evidence for TF-eQTL interactions falling into that TF's regulon. Large black dots depict overall enrichment across TFs. **C)** Enrichment for allele-specific TF binding (ASB) for TF-eQTL interactions with two lines of evidence. Shaded area contains statistics for unmatched TF ASB analysis. Below that, statistics for matched TF ASB analysis is shown, with TFs with more than one expected ASB event plotted individually, and all other TFs combined (other).

3.3.6 IRF1 knockdown validates IRF1-eQTL interactions

Our dual-evidence TF regulators included 58 eQTL effects putatively regulated by IRF1, which we assessed further with an IRF1 knockdown experiment. We used data from a CRISPR-interference-mediated knockdown of IRF1 in HEK293-TLR4 cells (Brandt, Kim-Hellmuth, et al. 2020) and measured genes' allele-specific expression (ASE) at knocked-down and control IRF1 levels [Fig. 3.4A,B]. A change in ASE between IRF1 conditions would suggest that IRF1 is regulating the effect of the heterozygous eQTL on gene expression.

We compared allele-specific gene expression in IRF1-knockdown and control cells, combining reads across all samples per condition to increase our power to discover differences in allelic expression. After filtering for sufficient coverage of a heterozygous coding SNP (>60 reads, >5% REF reads, >5% ALT reads, and <5% non-REF/ALT reads), we were left with 1,221 genes for which we performed Fisher's exact test for imbalanced allelic expression across conditions. A low Fisher's test p-value indicates that the two alleles are expressed at different ratios in the knockdown and control conditions, suggesting that IRF1 controls the expression of the gene in an allele-specific manner in this cell line.

We discovered 87 nominally significant genes with differing ASE between IRF1 conditions (Fisher's exact test $p < 0.05$). These genes were significantly enriched to overlap our previously discovered IRF1-eQTL genes (dual evidence TF-eQTLs OR = 8.03, Fisher's exact test $p = 0.015$) [Fig. 3.4C]. Of the dual-evidence TF-eQTL genes with measurable ASE, all seven were heterozygous for an implicated top IRF1-eQTL variant, thus we could expect all to show differing ASE between IRF1 conditions. Indeed, three genes, *ERI1*, *MYOM2*, and lncRNA *RP5-1092A3.4* were nominally significant, and all seven genes had p values in the lower quartile of tested genes, with a maximum p value of 0.31 [Fig. 3.4E; SFig. 14, 15]. Examining ASE in this IRF1 knockdown experiment validated 3/7 of our testable IRF1-eQTL interactions and demonstrates the high promise of this method to generate useful TF regulation information that can be applied to understand allele-specific regulation in new contexts.

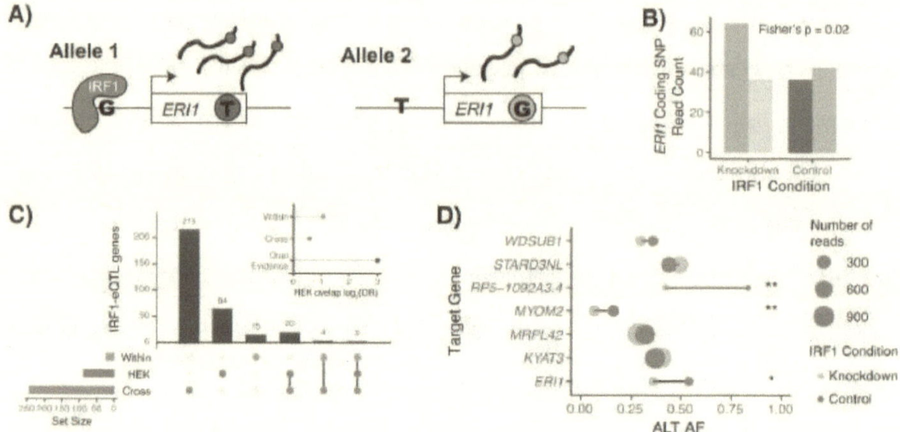

Figure 3.4: IRF1-eQTL interactions in HEK293-TLR4 IRF1 knockdown. A) Depiction of allele-specific expression, with IRF1 preferentially binding to the G-allele in the regulatory region of the *ERI1* target gene. This leads to higher expression of allele 1, which we can measure based on the presence of a heterozygous coding SNP in the *ERI1* transcript. **B)** Read counts for *ERI1* coding SNP alleles in both knockdown and control conditions. In this example, we observe allelic effects at lower (knockdown) IRF1 levels, while higher (control) levels of IRF1 may saturate binding to both alleles. Conditions are compared using Fisher's exact test of allelic counts. **C)** Sharing of IRF1-interacting eQTL genes in within-tissue (blue), cross-tissue expression-based (red), and HEK293 IRF1 knockdown (green) datasets. Inset shows enrichment for overlap between HEK293T IRF1-eQTL genes and listed datasets. **D)** HEK293 coding SNP alternative allele frequency in dual-evidence IRF1-eQTL genes that were heterozygous for a top TF-eQTL variant and had adequate coverage of a heterozygous coding SNP. * indicates a Fisher's p value < 0.05, ** < 0.01 of allelic counts vs. condition.

3.3.7 TF regulation of gene-by-environment effects and genetic effects on phenotype

We hypothesized that our TF-eQTLs could shed light on mechanisms of gene-by-environment (GxE) interactions that represent environmental conditions that affect genetic control of a phenotype, and altered TF level could be the mechanism by which the environmental condition regulates the genetic effects. In a recent large-scale study, Findley et al. tested the effects of 14 environmental treatments on allele-specific gene expression in three cell lines, discovering 979 genes with GxE effects, 850 of which were also found to have a GxE interaction by a previous study (Findley et al. 2021). We overlapped our dual evidence TF-eQTL genes with these replicated

GxE interacting genes and found 92 overlaps (OR = 2.67, Fisher's exact test $p = 1.4x10^{-14}$) [Fig. 3.5A], which offer potential direct mechanistic interpretations of the environmental effects on genetic control of gene expression [STable 3]. For instance, we found multiple GxE interactions for copper treatment that overlapped TF-eQTL genes for MITF or RELA; both TFs have been found to respond to copper exposure (McElwee, Song, and Freedman 2009; Hu Frisk et al. 2017), thus they could be the mechanism by which copper regulates genetic effects at these loci. Thus, combining TF-eQTL mechanisms with GxE interactions therefore has the potential to elucidate direct mechanisms of environmental effects.

We next assessed if we could use our TF-eQTLs to discover TF regulators of GWAS loci. Colocalization methods can combine statistical signals from eQTLs and GWAS loci to determine if the gene and phenotype regulation share a causal variant, implying that genetic regulation of the gene may be the causal mechanism of the genetic effect on phenotype. We obtained GWAS-eQTL colocalization data of GTEx eQTLs and 76 GWAS traits (Wen, Pique-Regi, and Luca 2017; Barbeira et al. 2021) and combined these with our dual-evidence TF-eQTLs. We saw that our TF-eQTL genes were more likely to colocalize with GWAS loci than all tested eQTL genes, with 27% of our TF-eQTL genes showing colocalization between a GWAS signal and an eQTL in any tissue and 9.5% showing colocalization between a GWAS signal and an eQTL in the same tissue where the TF-eQTL was discovered (OR = 2.00, 1.65, Fisher's exact test $p = 2.1x10^{-29}$, $1.1x10^{-10}$, respectively) [Fig. 3.5B]. We found 205 colocalizations between a GWAS signal and an eQTL signal in a tissue with a dual evidence TF-eQTL that had high LD between the lead colocalization and TF-eQTL variants ($r^2 > 0.4$), which represent potential TF regulators of genetic effects on phenotype [STable 3].

One example of this relationship is an *APBB1IP* eQTL that interacts with transcription factor IKZF1. This eQTL is present in 31 GTEx tissues and colocalized with GWAS signals for four red and white blood cell traits (ENLOC regional conditional probability > 0.5), suggesting that genetic control of these traits could be mediated by *APBB1IP* expression (Astle et al. 2016; Barbeira et al. 2021; Wen, Pique-Regi, and Luca 2017) [Fig. 3.5C; SFig. 16; STable 4]. We observed three tissues (pituitary gland, thyroid, and tibial artery) with TF-eQTL interactions for the *APBB1IP* gene with IKZF1 (Georgopoulos 2002; Ezzat et al. 2006) [Fig. 3.5D,E; SFig. 17]. Supporting IKZF1 regulation of this eQTL, the top TF-eQTL and GWAS variants were highly linked ($r^2 > 0.85$) to *rs1335540*, a SNP found 15 bases upstream of an *APBB1IP* transcript start site that overlaps an IKZF1 ChIP-seq peak and matches a IKZF1 motif (Kheradpour and Kellis 2014; Kulakovskiy et al. 2018; ENCODE Project Consortium et al. 2007) [Fig. 3.5F, SFig. 17, 18]. *APBB1IP* eQTLs in all three tissues with an IKZF1-eQTL interaction showed colocalization with blood cell traits. *APBB1IP* mediates blood cell adhesion and immune response (Patsoukis et al. 2017; Lagarrigue, Kim, and Ginsberg 2016). It is also involved in integrin-mediated changes in the actin cytoskeleton of mammalian cells (Lafuente et al. 2004; Lagarrigue et al. 2015) and its orthologue MIG-10 has been shown to regulate axon outgrowth in *C. elegans* neurons (Chang et al. 2006). IKZF1 is a chromatin-remodeling TF involved in lymphocyte development as well as the neuroendocrine system (Georgopoulos 2002; Ezzat et al. 2006). These findings offer two explanations for the genetic control of blood cell traits by *APBB1IP* expression: 1) via altered gene expression in the blood cells themselves, or 2) via neuroendocrine control of blood cell counts originating with altered gene expression in neurons. Offering further support to the neuroendocrine hypothesis, thyroid dysfunction has been shown to alter red and white blood cell counts (Irvine et al. 1977; Ahmed and Mohammed 2020), and the IKZF1-eQTL interactions were observed in neuroendocrine tissues. Regardless, given the shared genetic signal in multiple tissues, we can hypothesize that IKZF1 regulates both *APBB1IP* expression and the implicated blood traits, suggesting a TF regulator of a complex trait's genetic association.

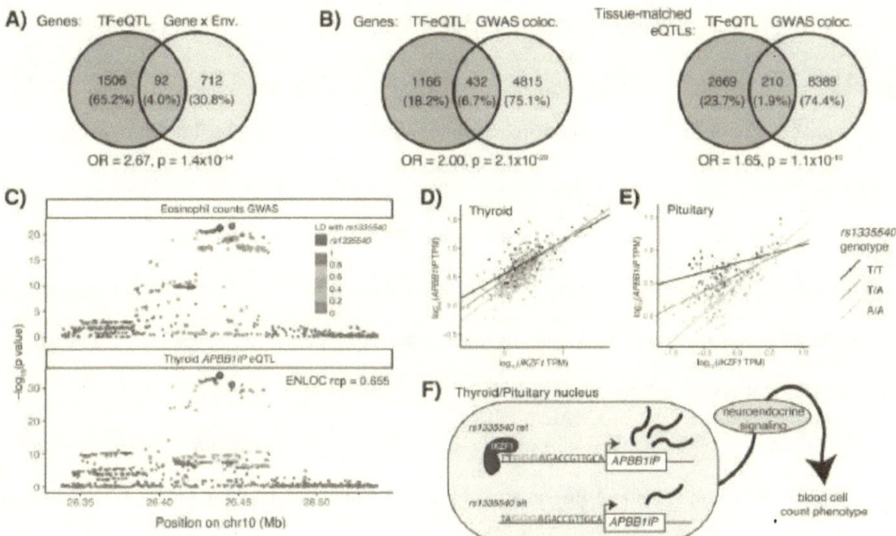

Figure 3.5: TF-eQTL implications for gene-by-environment and GWAS effects. A) Overlap of TF-eQTL genes with GxE genes from Findley et al. 2021. **B)** Overlap of TF-eQTL genes with GWAS colocalizing eQTL genes from GTEx. Left: overlap for a gene with a TF-eQTL in any tissue and colocalizing eQTL in any tissue. Right: overlap of tissue eQTLs with TF-eQTL and/or colocalizing GWAS locus in the given tissue. **C)** Representative eQTL and GWAS p-values are plotted for variants in the region of an *APBB1IP* eQTL and blood trait GWAS locus. Lead variants from IKZF1-eQTL interactions in thyroid, pituitary, and tibial artery are larger and outlined in black. (The lead variant from pituitary/artery cannot be seen as it falls behind rs1335540.) **D) & E)** Individual samples in thyroid and pituitary tissues are plotted by *IKZF1* and *APBB1IP* expression, and linear regression lines are plotted by genotype. The difference in APBB1IP expression between the genotypes gets smaller as *IKZF1* expression increases across the samples. **F)** Schematic of IKZF1 regulation of *APBB1IP* and blood cell counts. An IKZF1 binding site predicted by the HOCOMOCO IKZF1 motif lies nine bases upstream of *APBB1IP*'s transcription start site, which is disrupted by the alternative allele of *rs1335540*. Under our neuroendocrine signaling hypothesis, *APBB1IP* expression in neuroendocrine tissues goes on to alter system-wide neuroendocrine signaling, which would cause changes in blood cell counts. As IKZF1 appears to regulate the *APBB1IP* eQTLs in these tissues, it would follow that IKZF1 TF therefore may regulate the effect of this locus on blood cell counts.

3.4 Discussion

In this chapter, we used the natural variation of TFs across tissues and individuals to discover 6,262 TF-eQTL interactions across 1,598 genes, which represent putative TF-based mechanisms of genetic effects on gene expression. These TF-eQTLs were supported by at least two lines of evidence, including cross-tissue and/or within-tissue variation. They were enriched to overlap ChIP-seq peaks and fall into the regulon of the implicated TF, corroborating with orthogonal evidence that these eQTLs are regulated by the implicated TFs. Furthermore, analysis of an IRF1-knockdown experiment validated three out of seven testable IRF1-eQTLs. We see that TF-eQTL genes are more likely to colocalize with GWAS loci and overlap genes with gene-by-environment effects, and our example of IKZF1 regulation of an *APBB1IP* eQTL that colocalizes with GWAS signals for blood cell traits illustrates how our TF model can be used to discover likely TF regulators of GWAS effects.

Given the high number of possible causal genetic variants and putative regulatory mechanisms based on statistical fine-mapping and functional annotation overlap, it is clear that additional methods are needed to pinpoint causal variants and mechanisms of quantitative trait loci. Our method offers a new approach to discovering TF regulation of a genetic variant's effects, which can help us determine the eQTL's potential mechanism of action and explain its context variability. One major advantage to our method is its accessibility. While functional annotations were used to choose variants to test and to validate our results, the main discoveries of the model were powered by sample genotypes and gene expression levels – the same data available in most eQTL analyses. We leverage variation cross-tissues and within-tissues, which both have value for discovering TF regulators of eQTL effects, but especially the within-tissue TF interaction analysis is applicable to any eQTL data set even when a large number of different conditions may not be available.

Understanding TF regulation of an eQTL effect can allow us to focus functional fine-mapping efforts only on the implicated TF, hopefully narrowing the focus to one or a handful of variants that disrupt binding sites predicted by that TF's motif or show allele-specific binding in its ChIP-seq data. Unlocking these mechanisms allows us to eventually improve our understanding of the regulatory code of the genome and how human genetic variation perturbs that system. One clear application of our approach is for discovering and interpreting gene-by-environment (GxE) effects on gene expression and phenotype. While GxE interactions on human phenotype have been difficult to assess, GxE interactions in relation to gene expression have been studied under various contexts (Moyerbrailean et al. 2016; Kim-Hellmuth et al. 2017; Findley et al. 2021, 2019; Knowles et al. 2018, 2017; Taylor et al. 2018; Gutierrez-Arcelus et al. 2020). Overlapping these effects with TF-eQTLs as in our analysis, or even performing TF-eQTL analysis in the environmental exposure datasets themselves, provides mechanistic hypotheses of how environmental effects impact genetic control of gene expression and phenotype.

We were surprised by the lack of validation of TF-eQTLs discovered with cross-tissue protein levels, since protein measurements should reflect TF activity levels more accurately than expression measurements. However, the protein data had less power, from a smaller number of individuals and tissues than the expression data, and mass spectrometry may have more technical noise than expression quantifications from RNA-seq. Another promising option for TF measurement in the model is TF activity as predicted by target gene expression (Alvarez et al. 2016), which should account for translation rates, post-translational modifications, and subcellular localization effects on TF activity that expression measurements cannot capture. Initial analyses with this datatype did not yield strong results, but as activity estimates improve, the option should be revisited.

Though we saw enrichment for TF ChIP-seq peaks and allele-specific binding, our TF binding enrichments were quite modest. For instance, the TF ChIP-seq overlap enrichment statistic of 0.05 for dual-evidence TF-eQTLs means that we observed 0.05 more variants with ChIP-seq overlap per TF-eQTL gene than expected – or one additional overlap per twenty genes. Part of this may arise from the lack of ChIP-seq data from relevant tissue and cell type contexts that match the GTEx eQTL data. Nonetheless, it is likely that our dual-evidence TF-eQTLs likely contain false positives. One of the factors that may contribute to this is the correlated expression between TFs, which is difficult to fully account for. Another important factor is TF-eQTL correlations that may be caused by cell type composition (Kim-Hellmuth et al. 2020), such that an eQTL only found in a given cell type might be correlated with TFs that are highly expressed in that cell type even when the TF does not specifically regulate the eQTL. While some of our discovered TF-eQTLs may be false positives due to cell type variability, the ChIP-seq enrichments and IRF1 validation indicate that the applied filters successfully remove many of the major cell type composition effects. Altogether, we consider our 6,262 TF-eQTLs to represent regulatory variants with an indication of being regulated by the implicated TFs, but full validation will require additional work.

In summary, in addition to this catalog of potential TF regulators of eQTLs, we hope that our methods of comparing TF level with genetic variant effect can be applied in additional eQTL datasets, as well as for splicing QTLs and other molecular phenotypes. Our approach has the potential to implicate mechanisms for eQTL effects that vary across contexts without requiring additional datatypes or experiments, though its integration with other lines of evidence can further strengthen the insights, as shown in this study. Additionally, our method can improve functional fine-mapping efforts by highlighting TFs that may be regulating a locus, which can be further investigated with functional genomic data for that TF such as motif prediction or allele-specific binding data. We believe this TF-based framework of genetic variant effect variability can advance our understanding of QTL and GWAS mechanisms and their context variability, with great promise for understanding environmental interactions that impact genetic disease risk.

Chapter 4: Unraveling the mechanisms of *LIPA* locus effects on coronary artery disease[3]

4.1 Introduction

4.1.1 Coronary artery disease

Coronary artery disease (CAD), the most common type of heart disease in the United States, is caused by cholesterol plaque build-up in the coronary artery, the vessel that supplies blood to the heart (CDC 2021). These plaque build-ups cause the coronary artery to narrow, a process called atherosclerosis, which blocks blood flow to the heart muscles and can result in heart attack or heart failure (CDC 2021). Multiple genome wide association studies (GWASs) have been conducted on CAD in European, South Asian, East Asian, and multi-ethnic populations (CARDIoGRAMplusC4D Consortium et al. 2013; Coronary Artery Disease (C4D) Genetics Consortium 2011; Koyama et al. 2020; Matsunaga et al. 2020; Nelson et al. 2017; Nikpay et al. 2015; Schunkert et al. 2011; van der Harst and Verweij 2018; Webb et al. 2017; Wild et al. 2011). These studies have identified approximately 160 genetic loci that are associated with CAD risk.

CAD shows pleiotropy with other complex traits. One study found that 39% of CAD-associated loci were also associated with traditional cardiovascular risk factors, such as cholesterol levels, blood pressure, and BMI (Webb et al. 2017). Most of these traits had genetic effects in the

---

[3] The molecular biology experiments described in this chapter were performed by Fang Li and Hanrui Zhang. GTEx genetic and gene expression data and CARDIoGRAM C4D Coronary Artery Disease GWAS data, including colocalization analysis, were provided by the GTEx Consortium. All remaining analyses were performed by Elise Flynn.

same direction overall (i.e., increased CAD risk and increased cardiovascular measurement associated with the same allele), except for HDL cholesterol-associated loci which showed an opposite effect (Webb et al. 2017). Additionally, 2/14 LDL cholesterol-associated loci and 3/5 BMI-associated loci showed opposite effects (Webb et al. 2017). Using Mendelian randomization to dissect the pleiotropy of CAD-associated loci found similar results, finding that increased LDL cholesterol and triglyceride levels were associated with increased CAD risk, while increased HDL cholesterol levels were not associated with risk (White et al. 2016). Another GWAS-based study using associations of all common variants (minor allele frequency > 0.01) across the genome found positive genetic correlation between CAD and BMI (r=0.60) (Nikpay et al. 2015). These results suggest common genetic pathways between CAD and cardiovascular measurements, but they also highlight a large portion of loci that have no observed associations with traditional cardiovascular risk factors.

Table 4.1. Pleiotropy of coronary artery disease.

Study	Method	Trait	Direction vs. CAD risk
(Webb et al. 2017)	GWAS loci	LDL	same (12/14 loci)
(Webb et al. 2017)	GWAS loci	HDL	opposite
(Webb et al. 2017)	GWAS loci	triglycerides	same
(Webb et al. 2017)	GWAS loci	BMI	mixed (2/5 same, 3/5 opposite)
(White et al. 2016)	Mendelian randomization	LDL	same
(White et al. 2016)	Mendelian randomization	HDL	none
(White et al. 2016)	Mendelian randomization	triglycerides	same
(Nikpay, Turner, and McPherson 2018)	All common variants	BMI	same

4.1.1 *LIPA* locus in CAD

GWASs and candidate gene studies have identified a CAD-associated signal near the *LIPA* gene (IBC 50K CAD Consortium 2011; Nelson et al. 2017; Webb et al. 2017; Nikpay et al. 2015; Wild et al. 2011) [TABLE 4.2]. These five studies identified three variants in very high LD ($r^2 > 0.95$): *rs2246942*, *rs2246833*, and *rs1412444*. These variants fall in or near the *LIPA* transcript and have been previously identified to be associated with changes in *LIPA* gene expression levels in monocytes, such that increased monocyte *LIPA* expression and increased CAD risk are associated with the same allele (Wild et al. 2011).

Table 4.2. Lead CAD GWAS variants in *LIPA* locus.

Study	Method	Population	Lead *LIPA* locus variant(s)
(Wild et al. 2011)	GWAS	European; 2078 cases, 2953 controls	*rs1412444*, *rs2246833*
(IBC 50K CAD Consortium 2011)	Candidate gene	European and South Asian; 15,596 cases, 34,992 controls	*rs2246942*
(Webb et al. 2017)	GWAS	European and South Asian; 30,533 cases, 42.530 controls	*rs2246833*, *rs11203042*
(Nikpay et al. 2015)	GWAS	Multi-ethnic; ~185,000 CAD cases and controls	*rs1412444*
(Nelson et al. 2017)	GWAS	Multi-ethnic	*rs2246942*

The *LIPA* gene encodes lysosomal acid lipase (LAL) protein, an enzyme that hydrolyzes cholesteryl esters and triglycerides in the lysosome (H. Zhang 2018). Cholesteryl esters are enriched in LDL cholesterol, and once they are transported into the cell, LAL breaks these down to free cholesterol and fatty acids before they are further metabolized in the endoplasmic reticulum and eventually transported out of the cell (Chistiakov, Bobryshev, and Orekhov 2016) [FIG 4.1]. This process is extremely important to the generation of cholesterol plaques that cause atherosclerosis. Briefly, these plaques are believed to be initiated by the presence of macrophage foam cells, which are macrophage cells filled with high levels of cholesterols and lipids (Yu et al. 2013). Multiple genes in the macrophage cholesterol metabolism pathway have been shown to lead to the formation of foam cells and/or atherosclerosis, but a pathological role of LAL has not yet been characterized (Baldán et al. 2006; Chistiakov, Bobryshev, and Orekhov 2016; Dai et al. 2012; Fazio et al. 2001; Handberg et al. 2012; Igarashi et al. 2010; Ranalletta et al. 2006; Su et al. 2005).

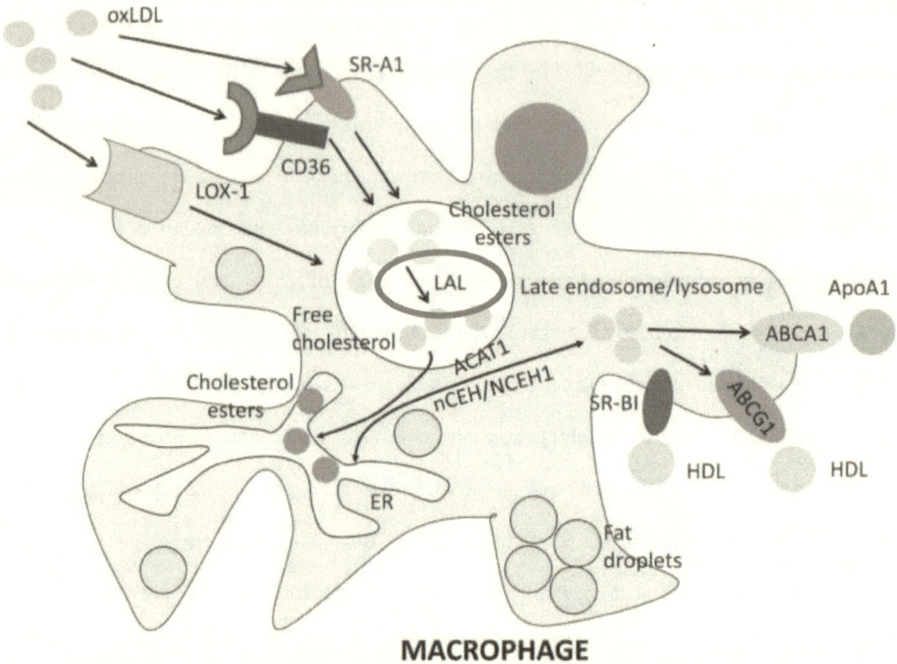

Figure 4.1: Macrophage cholesterol processing pathway. The role of LAL is highlighted in red in the middle of the diagram. LAL processes cholesterol esters into free cholesterol. Adapted from (Chistiakov, Bobryshev, and Orekhov 2016).

Lending further support to a macrophage-specific role of *LIPA* in CAD, the *LIPA* locus is not associated with other cardiometabolic traits including cholesterol, triglycerides, or BMI (IBC 50K CAD Consortium 2011; Webb et al. 2017; Wild et al. 2011; Willer et al. 2013). Interestingly, monocyte *LIPA* gene expression has been associated with lower HDL-cholesterol levels and impaired endothelial function, but this same study found no association with the lead CAD GWAS/*LIPA* eQTL variants (*rs1412444* and *rs2246833*) and any cardiometabolic traits (Wild et al. 2011). This suggests that the locus either 1) exerts its effects via a mechanism other than lowered gene expression, or 2) has a context-specific effect in macrophages, after they are differentiated from monocytes. Supporting the first option, a missense *LIPA* variant, *rs1051338*, is in very high LD ($r^2 = 0.86$) with *rs1412444*; however, it was found to have no functional effect on LAL activity (Evans et al. 2019). Thus, the functional mechanisms of the *LIPA* locus on CAD risk remain an open question.

4.1.3 Summary

In this chapter, we seek to characterize the functional mechanisms of the *LIPA* locus on CAD risk with statistical and functional fine-mapping of the *LIPA* eQTL. We find that a CAD GWAS signal colocalizes with *LIPA* eQTLs in multiple tissues, including Spleen and Whole Blood, and the lead SNP of the GWAS locus has eQTL effects in monocytes. We find enhancer effects of two variants, *rs141444* and *rs1320496*, in an experimental luciferase assay. These variants are in partial LD ($r^2 = 0.45$, D' = 1) and fall only 100 bases from each other, but we are able to see independent statistical effects of the two variants in the eQTL and GWAS data. Finally, we find evidence that PU.1 may regulate the effects of *rs1320496* on *LIPA* expression, offering a potential regulator of this locus's effects on gene expression and disease risk.

4.2 Materials and Methods

4.2.1 Datasets

One GWAS dataset (CARDIoGRAM C4D Coronary Artery Disease (Nikpay et al. 2015)) and two eQTL datasets (Genotype Tissue Expression (GTEx) v8 (GTEx Consortium 2020), Blueprint (L. Chen et al. 2016)) were used for our analyses. CARDIoGRAMplusC4D 1000

Genomes-based GWAS data consisted of a multi-ethnic meta-analysis of 60,801 CAD cases and 123,504 controls (Nikpay et al. 2015). Summary statistics were previously downloaded from the CARDIoGRAMplusC4D website and harmonized with GTEx variants by the GTEx Consortium. Briefly, GWAS results were lifted over to hg38, variants were matched between the two datasets, and z scores were imputed for missing variants using GTEx genotypes from European individuals (GTEx Consortium 2020; Barbeira et al. 2021).

GTEx v8 data were provided by the GTEx Consortium, including whole genome sequencing for 838 individuals and RNA sequencing from 15,201 samples across 49 tissues, as well as *cis*-eQTL calculations in each tissue (GTEx Consortium 2020). Blueprint eQTL summary statistics were downloaded from the WP10 Data Portal for all *LIPA* gene traits (L. Chen et al. 2016).

4.2.2 Colocalization

Colocalization between CAD GWAS loci and GTEx *LIPA* eQTLs was previously performed by the GTEx Consortium using ENLOC software (Wen, Pique-Regi, and Luca 2017; GTEx Consortium 2020; Barbeira et al. 2021). GTEx tissue gene expression levels and genotypes were processed with DAPG (Wen et al. 2016), and CAD GWAS variants were split into approximately LD-independent regions. ENLOC was run per region and per GTEx tissue to generate regional colocalization probabilities (rcp) that the GWAS locus and eQTL share a genetic effect (Wen, Pique-Regi, and Luca 2017).

4.2.3 TF-eQTL interactions

We correlated PU.1 expression levels with *LIPA* eQTL effects across GTEx tissues, as has been previously described (Flynn et al. 2021). For this analysis, we only analyzed 74 transcription factors and one variant per gene, that which was the lead CAVEMAN fine-mapped variant (Brown et al. 2017) in the GTEx tissue with the largest significant eQTL effect size as calculated by log2 allelic fold change (aFC) (Mohammadi et al. 2017b). We performed Benjamini-Hochberg multiple testing correction across all genes per transcription factor (Benjamini and Hochberg 1995).

4.2.4 Functional overlap of *LIPA*-/CAD-associated variants

The PU.1 motif was taken from ENCODE motifs (Kheradpour and Kellis 2014). PU.1 allele-specific binding at *rs1412445* was first discovered in AlleleDB (J. Chen et al. 2016). However, *rs1320496* was not tested in this dataset, as it is not found in 1000 Genomes. We found that the GM12891 LCL ENCODE PU.1 ChIP-seq sample was heterozygous for all three SNPs of interest (*rs1412444*, *rs1412445*, and *rs1320496*) (ENCODE Project Consortium et al. 2007), and we used the Integrative Genomics Viewer to count the reads aligned to each allele of each SNP (Robinson et al. 2011).

4.2.5 Independent effects of *LIPA*-/CAD-associated variants

In order to disentangle the effects of variants in high LD, we used various linear regression models to estimate the SNPs' independent effects on both LIPA gene expression and CAD. Since *rs1412444* and *rs1412445* were in almost perfect LD in both GTEx and CARDIoGRAM C4D cohorts, we included only *rs1412445* in our models (G_P) as well as *rs1320496* (G_G).

For LIPA eQTL analysis, we fit four linear models:

rs1412445 only: $E = \beta_R G_R + \beta_C cov + \varepsilon$ (Eq 4.1)

rs1320496 only: $E = \beta_G G_G + \beta_C cov + \varepsilon$ (Eq 4.2)

Interaction model: $E = \beta_R G_R + \beta_G G_G + \beta_{RG} G_R * G_G + \beta_C\, cov + \varepsilon$ (Eq 4.3)

Conditional model: $E - \widehat{\beta_R^1} * G_R = \beta_G G_G + \beta_C cov + \varepsilon$ (Eq 4.4)

where E is log2-transformed LIPA gene count data normalized with deseq2 (Love, Huber, and Anders 2014); G_R and G_G are alternative allele dosages for *rs1412445* and *rs1320496*, respectively; and *cov* are the covariates used by GTEx for eQTL discovery including genotype principal components, sequencing information, donor sex, and Probabilistic Estimation of Expression Residuals (PEER) method factors (Stegle et al. 2010; GTEx Consortium 2020). For the conditional model, we used from the *rs1412445* only model to remove the effect of *rs1412444/rs1412445* on expression, and a linear model using rs1320496 was fit to the residual expression.

For CAD GWAS analysis, we used individual SNP beta estimates and p-values as reported in the summary statistics. We calculated the conditional effect of *rs1320496* on CAD (conditional on *rs1412445*) using the cojo tool from the GCTA software package (Yang et al. 2011; Z. Zhu et al. 2018). GCTA was run with CAD GWAS summary statistics, GTEx genotypes for LD structure, and *rs1412445* as a conditional SNP.

4.2.6 Luciferase assay

To functionally identify the regulatory region of control of *LIPA* expression, we constructed plasmids of human LIPA sequence in *rs1412444* region (hg19_dna range= chr10:91002499-91003138) and *rs2246833* region (hg19_dna range=chr10:91005571-91006002). These regions were amplified and cloned into KpnI and XhoI restriction sites of pGL4.23 vector (Promega, E8411) to generate pGL4.23-*rs1412444*-region and pGL4.23-

rs2246833-region plasmids. The cloned fragments were *confirmed* by Sanger Sequencing. Primers used for plasmid construction were listed as: *rs1412444* region, 5'-ATATATGGTACCTTTCTGTTAGTATACGAGGAGCC-3'; anti-*rs1412444* region, 5'-ATATATCTCGAGCAGTGGGGAGTCTTCAAGGA-3'; *rs2246833* region, 5'-ATATATGGTACC CAGTCTCCCACATTAACAAGCA-3'; and anti-*rs2246833* region, 5'-ATATATCTCGAGCCAGCAGGGGATCTCTCAAA-3'.

To further identify the causal variants in *LIPA rs1412444* region, we performed site-directed mutagenesis. Cytosine at SNPs of *rs1412444*, *rs1320496*, and *rs1412445* were replaced as thymidine with QuickChange II XL Site-Directed Mutagenesis Kit (Agilent, #200521) following manufacturer's instructions. Primers used to each SNP were designed as: *rs1412445*, 5'-GGTCATTAGGAGGATGTTGGTGCTATTAATAATAGAGGAGG-3'; anti-*rs1412445*, 5'-CCTCCTCTATTATTAATAGCACCAACATCCTCCTAATGACC-3'; *rs1320496*, 5'-GGAGGGGAAGTGGGATGCATG-3'; anti-*rs1320496*, 5'-CATGCATCCCACTTCCCCTCC-3'; *rs1412444*, 5'- GCCTTTAAACACTGGAAATAACACCAGTGGC-3'; and anti-*rs1412444*, 5'- GCCACTGGTGTTATTTCCAGTGTTTAAAGGC-3'. The obtained fragments were cloned into sites of KpnI/ XhoI in pGL4.23 vector and confirmed by Sanger sequencing. pGL4.23-CCC was referred to as plasmids containing *LIPA rs1412444* region without mutations. pGL4.23-CTC was referred to as plasmids containing the risk allele of SNP *rs1320496* in *rs1412444* region. pGL4.23-TTT represented plasmids containing risk alleles of all three SNPs in *rs1412444* region. These three plasmids resembled three haplotypes identified in human subjects.

To detect enhancer activity in the luciferase reporter assay, constructed pGL4.23 plasmids containing risk regions or alleles (500 ng) were individually mixed with 10 ng of pGL4.73 Renilla vector (Promega, E6911) and co-transfected to THP-1 monocytes or HEK cells through electroporation (Lonza, V4XC-3024). After 24 hours, cells were lysed and subjected to luciferase activity assay using Dual-Luciferase Assay System (Promega, E1960). The results were expressed as the ratio of firefly luciferase activity over Renilla luciferase activity.

4.3 Results

4.3.1 *LIPA* eQTLs and CAD colocalization

GWAS-eQTL colocalization is a commonly used method to implicate causal genes underlying a genetic association with disease. Significant *LIPA* eQTLs are observed in multiple GTEx tissues, with the largest effects in Whole Blood and Spleen (GTEx Consortium 2020) [FIG 4.2A], as well as in monocyte, neutrophil, and T-cell cell lines in Blueprint (L. Chen et al. 2016) [FIG 4.2B]. Colocalization analysis performed by the GTEx Consortium with ENLOC software (Wen, Pique-Regi, and Luca 2017; GTEx Consortium 2020; Barbeira et al. 2021) revealed high regional colocalization probabilities for CARDIoGRAM C4D CAD GWAS signal and *LIPA* eQTLs in both Whole Blood and Spleen (rcp = 0.66, 0.76, respectively) [FIG 4.3], indicating that CAD risk and *LIPA* gene expression likely share a genetic regulatory signal. *LIPA* was the closest and the only colocalizing gene in the region in these two tissues [FIG 4.4]. Colocalization with Blueprint eQTLs was not available, but monocytes are the only cell type with a significant eQTL for the lead CAD GWAS variant (*rs1412444*), supporting previous findings that monocytes may be the causal cell type for the genetic effect of this locus on coronary artery disease. These findings suggest that genetic control of CAD risk at this locus could be mediated by *LIPA* expression, especially in blood and immune cell types related to monocytes.

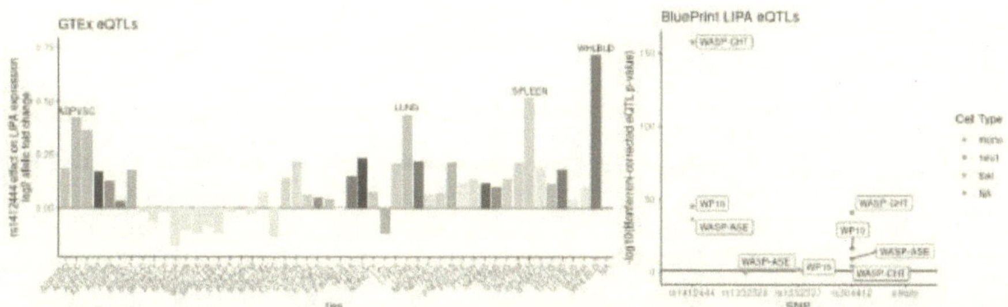

Figure 4.2: LIPA eQTLs. (Left) *LIPA* eQTL effect size of rs1412444 across GTEx tissues. Tissues with largest effect sizes are written. (Right) *LIPA* eQTL significance in BluePrint cell types based on various eQTL detection methods.

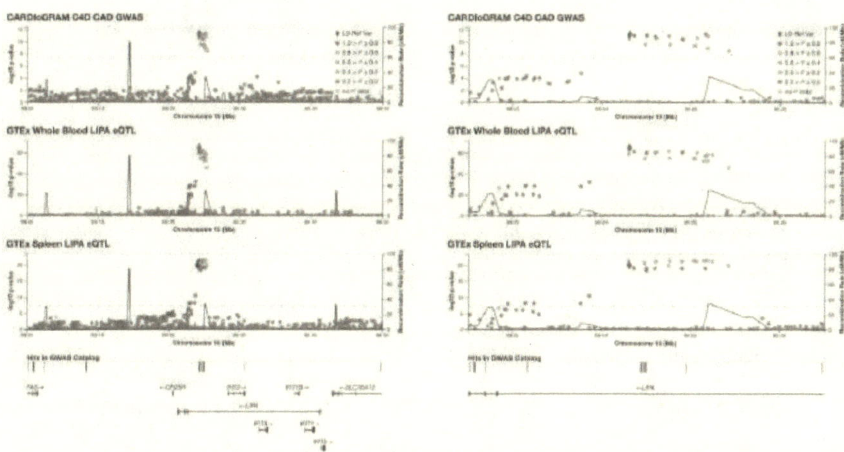

Figure 4.3: LocusZoom plots of Coronary Artery Disease GWAS and GTEx *LIPA* eQTLs. Height indicates strength (-log10(p value)) of variant's association with the phenotype, and the linkage with the top GWAS SNP (*rs1412444*) is shown by dot color. All three datasets show a similar p-value landscape, confirmed by ENLOC colocalization analysis, indicating that they may share a genetic signal. *LIPA* is the closest and the only colocalizing gene in the region.

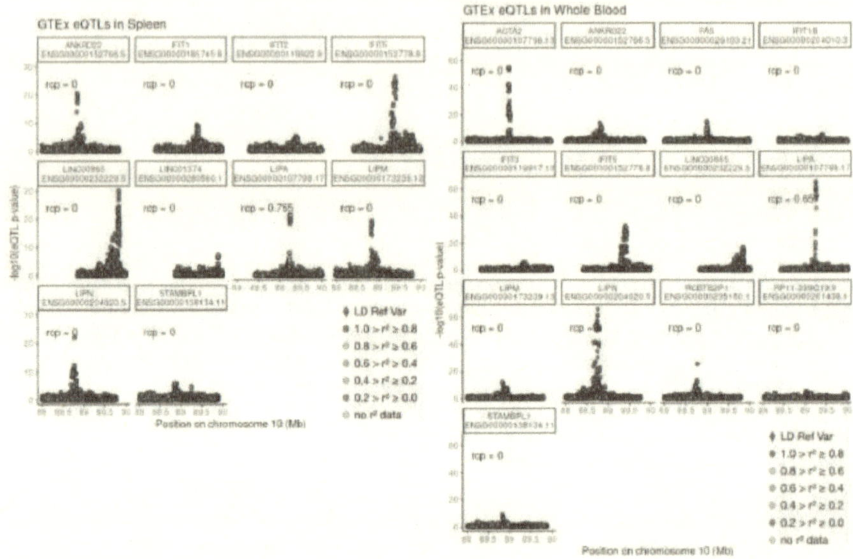

Figure 4.4: Spleen and Whole Blood eQTLs in GWAS signal region. Height indicates strength (-log10(p value)) of variant's association with gene expression, and the linkage with the top GWAS SNP (*rs1412444*) is shown by dot color. *LIPA* is the only gene with an ENLOC regional conditional probability (rcp) greater than 0.

4.3.2 Independent variant effects

Though there are many variants in high LD with *rs1412444*, the lead variant of the CAD GWAS locus, we observed that the specific region of *rs1412444* showed enhancer activity in monocytes [FIG 4.6]. Thus, we examined the three variants of interest in this region: *rs1412445*, *rs1320496*, and *rs1412444*. These variants fall within 150 bases of each other. *rs1412444* and *rs1412445* are in extremely high LD ($r^2 = 0.99$ in GTEx), while *rs1320496*, the lead variant of the *LIPA* eQTL in Spleen, is partially linked ($r^2 = 0.44$ in GTEx). A luciferase expression assay of all possible haplotypes of these three variants showed transcriptional effects of *rs1412445* and *rs1320496* individually, but no effect of *rs1412444* [FIG 4.7A]. Combinatorial effects of the variants are more difficult to assess. However, follow up of the three haplotypes regularly observed in the human population (CCC, CTC, and TTT), showed incremental effects of *rs1320496* and *rs1412444/rs1412445* on gene expression (ps < 0.05) [FIG 4.7B]. These experimental results suggest that *rs1320496* and *rs1412445* can exert independent effects on gene expression, and we next examined if there was statistical evidence that these two variants exert independent effects on gene expression and disease risk in population association studies.

We examined the effect of *rs1320496* and *rs1412445* individually and in combination on Whole Blood *LIPA* expression levels and on CAD prevalence. This analysis is complicated by the high LD ($r^2 = 0.45$, D' = 1) of the two SNPs in the population, but we used interaction models and conditional analysis to disentangle the individual SNP effects. Each SNP had significant associations with both *LIPA* expression and with CAD risk individually (eQTL ps < 10^{-59}, GWAS ps < 10^{-10}), and both SNPs had a significant association in an interaction model of *LIPA* expression (ps < 10^{-11}) [FIG 4.8]. Most importantly, *rs1320496* still has significant associations with both LIPA expression and CAD once the entire effect of *rs1412445* is removed from the data (eQTL p = 3×10^{-10}, GWAS p = 0.03; see *Methods* for more detail) [FIG 4.8]. These statistical modeling results, combined with the experimental effects of the SNPs in the luciferase assays, suggest that both *rs1412445* and *rs1320496* exert independent effects on *LIPA* expression and on CAD risk and support the presence of multiple causal variants at this locus.

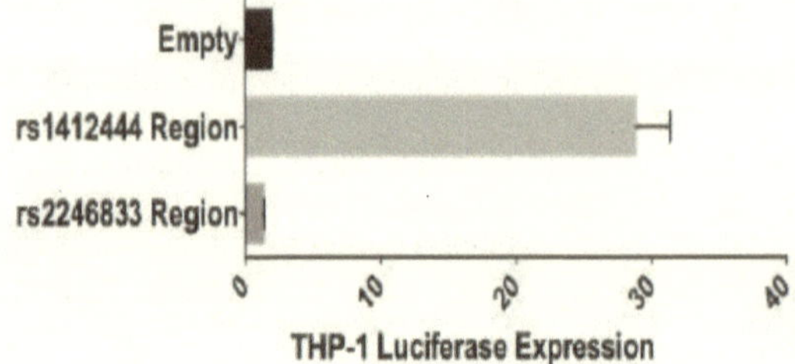

Figure 4.6: Luciferase assay of putative regulatory regions. Luciferase expression in THP-1 monocytes is plotted for two fine-mapped GWAS regions. *rs1412444* region shows expression activity, while *rs2246833* does not.

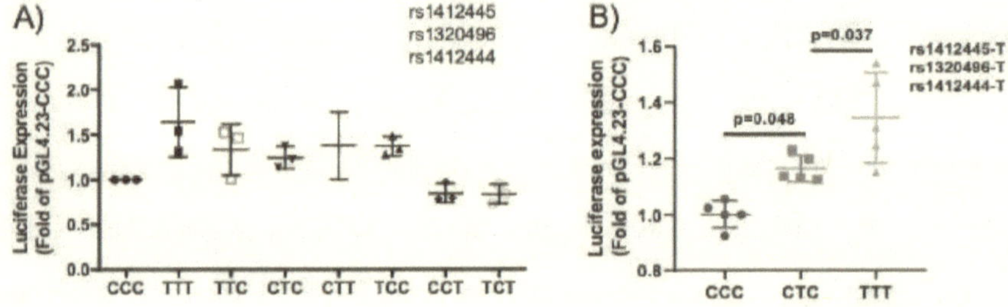

Figure 4.7: Luciferase assay of allelic effects of *LIPA*/CAD variants. A) Luciferase expression is plotted for all possible haplotype combinations of *rs1412445*, *rs1320496*, and *rs1412444*. All haplotypes with alternative alleles for *rs1412445* and *rs1320496* appear to show increased gene expression versus the all-reference haplotype. **B)** Luciferase expression for additional replicates of common population haplotypes of *rs1412445*, *rs1320496*, and *rs1412444*. The all-alternative haplotype has nominally significantly higher expression than the haplotype with only *rs1320496* alternative, which has nominally significantly higher expression than the all-reference haplotype.

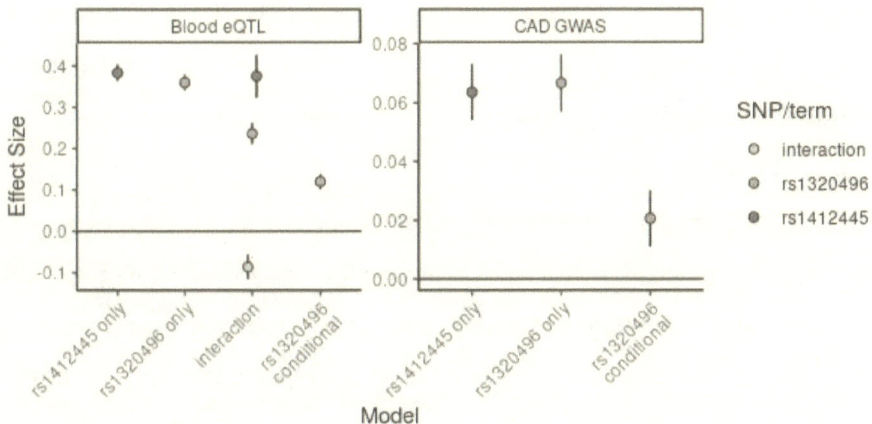

Figure 4.8: Conditional analysis of SNPs of interest. Since both rs1412445 and rs1320496 showed enhancer activity in the luciferase assay, we examined the effect of the two SNPs individually and in combination on Blood LIPA expression levels and CAD prevalence. The effect size (regression coefficient, or beta) of the SNP is shown on the y-axis, with different linear models along the x-axis. Black lines represent standard deviation. Each SNP has significant associations with both LIPA expression and with CAD individually (rs1412445 only and rs1320496 only; eQTL ps<10^-59, GWAS ps<10^-10), and both SNPs have a significant association in an interaction model of LIPA expression (interaction; ps<10^-11). Most importantly, rs1320496 still has significant associations with both LIPA expression and CAD once the entire effect of rs1412445 is removed from the data (rs1320496 conditional; eQTL p=3*10^-10, GWAS p=0.03; see Methods for more detail).

4.3.3 PU.1 regulation of *rs1320496*

Many eQTLs are expected to affect gene expression by disrupting transcription factor binding, though few transcription factor mechanisms of eQTLs have been directly validated. As described in Chapter 3, transcription factor regulators of regulatory variant effects can be hypothesized using transcription factor variation across and within contexts. To this end, we investigated transcription factor - *LIPA* eQTL relationships across 49 GTEx tissues, for all top *LIPA* eQTL variants in any GTEx tissue. We observed significant correlations between nine transcription factors and cross-tissue eQTL effects of *rs1320496*; the strongest and most significant effect was observed for PU.1, encoded by the *SPI1* gene (Spearman rho = 0.57, p =

$5.8x10^{-5}$) [FIG 4.9]. PU.1 is a transcription factor involved in hematopoiesis, including the differentiation of monocytes into macrophages (DeKoter, Walsh, and Singh 1998; Tagore et al. 2015), thus the *LIPA* eQTL's high activity in blood, spleen, and monocytes could be explained by this transcription factor.

We next examined transcription factor binding site information at this locus. Many transcription factor ChIP-seq peaks overlap the three SNPs in the region, including PU.1 [FIG 4.10], and we saw that the alternative allele of *rs1320496* (T) is predicted to strengthen the motif-based predicted binding of PU.1. We then examined allele-specific binding (ASB) of PU.1 ENCODE ChIP-seq reads, with the premise that an allelic imbalance in the ChIP-seq reads would suggest that a variant in the locus was disrupting PU.1 binding *in vivo*. We observed that all three variants showed allelic imbalance, with higher levels of the motif-matching alternative T allele present in the ChIP-seq reads [FIG 4.11]. *rs1412445* showed significant imbalance in the AlleleDB dataset (J. Chen et al. 2016). (*rs1320496* was not tested.) Though we can't differentiate between the three variants in ChIP-seq binding data due to their proximity, *rs1320496* was the only variant predicted to disrupt a PU.1 binding site. Combined with the cross-tissue pattern of PU.1 levels and *rs1320496 LIPA* eQTL effects, these results suggest that *rs1320496* exerts its effect on LIPA expression (and potentially CAD) via altered PU.1 binding.

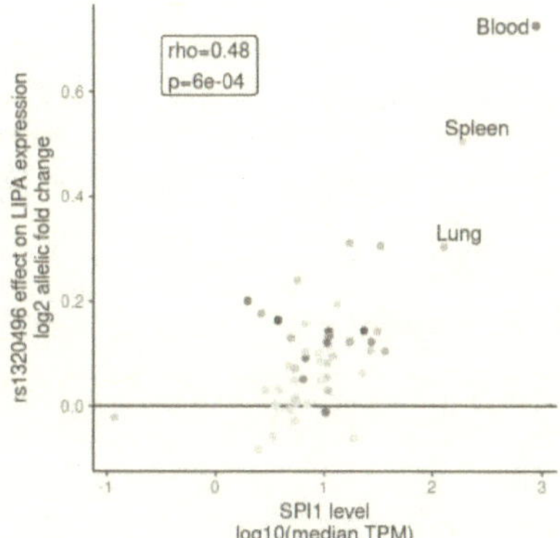

Figure 4.9: Relationships between transcription factor level and eQTL effect sizes across tissues. *rs1320496 LIPA* eQTL effect size (log2 allelic fold change) vs. *SPI1* level (log10(median transcripts per million in tissue)) across GTEx tissues. eQTL effect sizes increase as *SPI1* level increases (Spearman rho=0.48, p=6*10^-4), suggesting PU.1 binding may influence the eQTL effect.

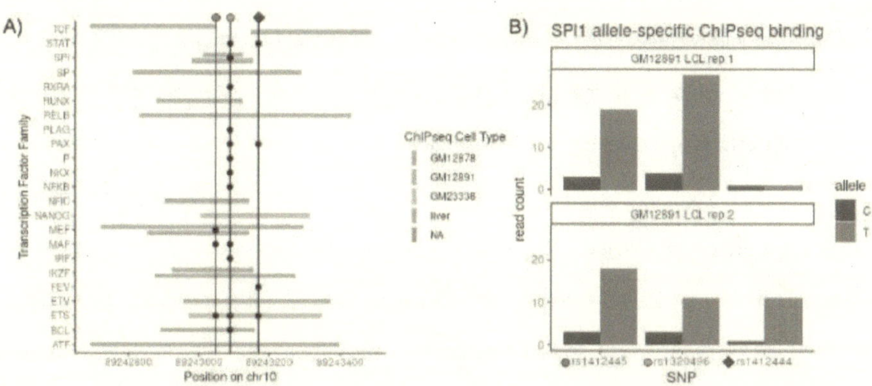

Figure 4.10: Transcription factor binding of *rs1320496* region. A) ENCODE TF ChIP-seq peaks (bars) are shown for the ~400 base pair flanking region of the SNPs of interest, while ENCODE TF motif disruptions (black dots) are shown for the three SNPs (*rs1412445* – red dot, *rs1320496* – green dot, *rs1412444* – purple diamond). TFs are organized by family instead of specific TF due to motif similarity within a family. Many TFs have some overlap in this region, and three TF families have both an overlapping ENCODE ChIP-seq peak and motif: SPI, MEF, ETS, and BCL. **B)** Allele-specific transcription factor ChIP-seq binding. Two TFs showed allele-specific binding (ASB) patterns in published TF ChIP-seq datasets (AlleleDB, ADASTRA). Count of SPI1 ChIP-seq reads aligned to reference (C, blue) and alternative (T, red) alleles in ENCODE SPI1 ChIP-seq conducted in LCL cell line. All three SNPs appear to show ASB, and rs1412445 was tested in AlleleDB and showed significant ASB.

4.4 Discussion

Our analyses have offered insight into functional mechanisms of the *rs1412444* locus on *LIPA* gene expression and coronary artery disease. We have prioritized two variants (*rs1412445*, *rs1320496*) with observed independent effects on gene expression and disease risk and have suggested a PU.1 transcription factor mechanism for *rs1320496*'s effects. Followup studies investigating the role of macrophage *LIPA* expression in CAD are ongoing but offer much promise for disentangling this locus's unique effects on disease risk.

One exciting angle of our current analysis is the applicability of our previously described transcription factor vs. eQTL effect approach for unraveling mechanisms of genetic control of complex traits (Flynn et al. 2021). Our analysis of PU.1 vs *LIPA* eQTLs prioritized the *rs1320496* variant, leading to discovery of its independent effects on gene expression and disease risk. Prior analyses had not investigated the variant as it was only in partial LD with the lead GWAS variant. Though further validation of the role of PU.1 is ongoing, the approach succeeded in helping to untangle the effects of a complex regulatory region.

Another exciting angle is the presence of multiple potentially causal variants with independent effects in a single GWAS locus. Though *rs1412444* and *rs1320496* were only in partial LD ($r^2 = 0.48$, D' = 1) and showed independent signals when analyzed, the conditional effects of *rs1320496* were not strong enough to have been discovered in a gene-wide or genome-wide analysis. Linked variants' independent effects can be dissected using functional annotations and experimental approaches, but examples of multiple validated causal variants in a single locus have been incredibly sparse (D.-L. Zhu et al. 2018; Sobreira et al. 2021). Recently, researchers used massively parallel reporter assays to determine which variants in linked variant sets were causal across thousands of eQTL loci (Abell et al. 2021). Quite strikingly, they found that 18% of all tested loci had more than one variant with a significant effect on expression, and 39% of all loci with at least one significant variant effect had multiple, and they found that multi-variant eQTLs were more likely to co-localize with GWAS loci (Abell et al. 2021). These recent findings suggest that future analyses will discover more GWAS loci with multiple causal variants, but we are happy to propose one of the first examples, to our knowledge.

Conclusion

Gene expression is regulated by local genomic sequence, and researchers have identified thousands of common genetic variants in the human population that associate with changes in gene expression. Many of these expression quantitative trait loci (eQTLs) lie in noncoding regions of the genome for which we have limited functional knowledge, impeding our ability to determine their mechanisms of action. Though general patterns of eQTL mechanisms have been researched, such as their enrichment in promoters, enhancers, and 5' and 3' untranslated regions, individual mechanisms of eQTL effects on gene expression remain largely unknown. Adding another layer of complexity, eQTLs have been assayed across tissues and under various environmental conditions, but the full range of eQTL activity is not known and is often context specific.

In this book, we explored the genetic regulatory landscape of gene expression across tissues and individuals in order to understand genetic variants' mechanisms of actions and context specificity. In Chapter 2, we investigated cross-tissue eQTL and gene expression patterns, including for GWAS genes. We found that eQTL effects show increasing, decreasing, and non-monotonic relationships with gene expression levels across tissues and that GWAS genes showed higher gene expression and larger eQTL effect sizes in relevant tissues for the GWAS trait. In Chapter 3, we used the natural variation of transcription factor activity among tissues and between individuals to elucidate mechanisms of action of eQTL regulatory variants and understand context specificity of eQTL effects. We discovered thousands of potential transcription factor mechanisms of eQTL effects, and we investigated the transcription factors' roles with orthogonal datasets and experimental approaches. Finally, in Chapter 4, we focused on a locus implicated in coronary artery disease risk and unraveled the causal variants and functional mechanisms of the locus's effects on gene expression and disease. We confirmed the locus's colocalization with an eQTL for the *LIPA* gene, and using statistical, functional, and experimental approaches, we highlighted two potential causal variants in partial linkage disequilibrium.

A central theme of our work is our model of transcription factor binding effects [FIG 3.1]. This model was supported by the differences in eGene expression between positively and negatively correlated eQTLs and the presence of non-monotonic patterns in Chapter 2. While we did not extensively investigate correlation directions and transcription factor levels in Chapter 3, we observed both positive and negative correlations. Finally, in Chapter 4, we demonstrated the usefulness of our model by predicting the PU.1 regulation of a *LIPA* eQTL and discovering *rs1320496*, a genetic variant with potential independent causal effects on *LIPA* gene expression and coronary artery disease risk. This theoretical transcription factor-based framework can be used to propose mechanisms for regulatory variant effects as well as to understand their context variability.

An ongoing challenge highlighted by our results is the difficulty in fine-mapping variants and determining their regulatory mechanisms. Many variants in a locus may show statistically significant associations with gene expression or phenotype, and we cannot reliably assume that the variant with the lowest p-value is the causal variant. Statistical fine-mapping can select a set of potentially causal variants with some probability, but these sets are often large – indeed, we saw that 44% of common variants in GTEx were in a fine-mapped eQTL set in at least one tissue. Once a variant set is statistically fine-mapped, functional annotations and experimental approaches can be used to determine causal variants, but the vast majority of molecular mechanisms of individual eQTLs or GWAS loci remain unknown. Adding a layer of complexity, multiple variants in the same locus can be causal, such as we discovered with our coronary artery disease and *LIPA* eQTL locus, and recent results suggest that this may happen quite often (Abell et al. 2021; Mouri et al. 2021).

We hope that our transcription factor-based approach can be applied by others to determine relevant transcription factor(s) driving eQTL mechanisms, which can then be used to inform fine-mapping and determine causal genetic variants that are predicted to bind the implicated transcription factor. The current approach to determine causal genetic variants and their functional mechanisms generally consists of statistically fine-mapping a locus, investigating genomic annotations overlapping the fine-mapped variants, and performing functional experiments of the variants' effects on gene expression. Our transcription factor analysis could allow researchers to fine-tune their genomic annotation investigations, focusing on variants that overlap annotations for the relevant transcription factor instead of the high percentage of variants that overlap any functional annotation. It could also inform follow-up experimental approaches, such as ensuring that the experimental cell line expresses the putative regulatory transcription factor. On its own, our transcription factor-based approach cannot provide conclusive evidence for a fine-mapped variant or its mechanism, but it adds a valuable layer of evidence to those available with the current genomics toolkit.

Another application of our transcription factor-based framework is to predict regulatory variant activity in new contexts. Variant effect predictors for coding effects have existed for many years (Ng and Henikoff 2001; Adzhubei et al. 2010; McLaren et al. 2016) and can predict deleterious effects of variants on protein structure and function. On the noncoding side, transcription factor binding models are a form of variant effect prediction (Kheradpour and Kellis 2014; Rastogi et al. 2018; Kulakovskiy et al. 2018), and convolutional neural network models have been developed to predict genetic effects on chromatin accessibility, transcription factor binding, and histone marks across contexts (Zhou and Troyanskaya 2015; Kelley, Snoek, and Rinn 2016). Recently, eQTL activity was predicted between tissues using variant, gene expression, and chromatin state annotations (GTEx Consortium 2020). However, these methods depend on transcription factor binding, chromatin accessibility, or other epigenomic data in the relevant context, as well as suffering from individual drawbacks for each method. While it would be naïve to expect that eQTL activity can be perfectly predicted from an eGene's expression or a single transcription factor's level, this framework could be integrated into existing models and has the benefit of requiring only gene expression data from the relevant context.

Of course, our research does not come without its limitations. Firstly, while our model is based on non-monotonic relationships between eQTL effects and transcription factor levels, we have not actually discovered any. Our discoveries in Chapter 2 of non-monotonic relationships between eQTL effects and eGene expression levels were based on limited datapoints (49 tissues), and upon closer examination many examples did not hold up. We did not perform extensive analysis of correlation direction for our transcription factor-eQTLs in Chapter 3, though initial analyses did discover both increasing and decreasing interactions. Secondly, cell type complications plagued multiple parts of our analysis. In Chapter 3, it was difficult to disentangle cell type interactions from our transcription factor-eQTL interactions, and our approach of removing tissues with large cell type variability did nothing to account for cell type interactions from the remaining tissues. We also likely suffered from the lack of transcription factor ChIP-seq data in relevant cell types when validating our model, highlighting a need for the genomic research community. Finally, in Chapter 4, the PU.1 ChIP-seq data was assayed in lymphoblastoid cell lines and our experiments were mainly conducted in THP-1, a monocyte-like cell line. However, previous research has suggested that the coronary artery disease locus effects on *LIPA* expression may be specific to macrophages, though monocytes are closely related. These issues again highlight the importance of conducting assays in the relevant context, as we do not yet fully understand the context variability of genetic variant effects.

Our current approach can be expanded and applied in many ways. In this book, we used transcription factor expression levels as a proxy for transcription factor activity. We were surprised by the lack of validation of transcription factor-eQTLs discovered with transcription factor protein levels, but this may be due to mass spectrometry's reduced resolution at the lower levels observed for transcription factors. Another promising option for future research is transcription factor activity as predicted by target gene expression (Alvarez et al. 2016), which should account for translation rates, post-translational modifications, and subcellular localization effects on transcription factor activity that expression measurements cannot capture. Our transcription factor model can also be applied for other types of regulatory factors and allelic phenotypes, such as RNA binding proteins and gene expression and transcript structure or long noncoding RNAs and gene expression. Long noncoding RNAs may have the added benefit of being more accurately assayed by RNA-seq, as they are not translated and are generally active in their transcribed state.

Our research provides a deeper understanding of gene regulation and of genetic and environmental contributions to complex traits and disease, enabling future research surrounding the context variability of genetic effects on gene expression and disease. Unraveling the context variability of eQTLs can help us determine the biological contexts in which GWAS loci affect human phenotype and disease, which has great implications for understanding disease etiology and for targeting pharmaceutical interventions. Determining eQTL mechanisms can also help us understand the non-coding genetic regulatory code, which informs gene expression throughout our bodies but still largely remains a mystery. We hope that our work will allow researchers to develop stronger functional genomic models and discovery tools and will contribute to a greater understanding of the context variability of genetic variant effects in the years to come.

References

1. Abell, Nathan S., Marianne K. DeGorter, Michael Gloudemans, Emily Greenwald, Kevin S. Smith, Zihuai He, and Stephen B. Montgomery. 2021. “Multiple Causal Variants Underlie Genetic Associations in Humans.” *BioRxiv*. https://doi.org/10.1101/2021.05.24.445471.

2. Abramov, Sergey, Alexandr Boytsov, Daria Bykova, Dmitry D. Penzar, Ivan Yevshin, Semyon K. Kolmykov, Marina V. Fridman, et al. 2021. “Landscape of Allele-Specific Transcription Factor Binding in the Human Genome.” *Nature Communications* 12 (1): 2751.

3. Adzhubei, Ivan A., Steffen Schmidt, Leonid Peshkin, Vasily E. Ramensky, Anna Gerasimova, Peer Bork, Alexey S. Kondrashov, and Shamil R. Sunyaev. 2010. “A Method and Server for Predicting Damaging Missense Mutations.” *Nature Methods* 7 (4): 248–49.

4. Aguirre-Gamboa, Raúl, Niek de Klein, Jennifer di Tommaso, Annique Claringbould, Monique Gp van der Wijst, Dylan de Vries, Harm Brugge, et al. 2020. “Deconvolution of Bulk Blood EQTL Effects into Immune Cell Subpopulations.” *BMC Bioinformatics* 21 (1): 243.

5. Ahmed, Sawer Sabri, and Ayad Ahmad Mohammed. 2020. “Effects of Thyroid Dysfunction on Hematological Parameters: Case Controlled Study.” *Annals of Western Medicine and Surgery* 57 (September): 52–55.

6. Akhtar, M. Waseem, Mi-Sung Kim, Megumi Adachi, Michael J. Morris, Xiaoxia Qi, James A. Richardson, Rhonda Bassel-Duby, Eric N. Olson, Ege T. Kavalali, and Lisa M. Monteggia. 2012. “In Vivo Analysis of MEF2 Transcription Factors in Synapse Regulation and Neuronal Survival.” *PloS One* 7 (4): e34863.

7. Alasoo, Kaur, Julia Rodrigues, John Danesh, Daniel F. Freitag, Dirk S. Paul, and Daniel J. Gaffney. 2019. “Genetic Effects on Promoter Usage Are Highly Context-Specific and Contribute to Complex Traits.” *ELife* 8 (January). https://doi.org/10.7554/eLife.41673.

8. Alasoo, Kaur, Julia Rodrigues, Subhankar Mukhopadhyay, Andrew J. Knights, Alice L. Mann, Kousik Kundu, HIPSCI Consortium, Christine Hale, Gordon Dougan, and Daniel J. Gaffney. 2018. “Shared Genetic Effects on Chromatin and Gene Expression Indicate a Role for Enhancer Priming in Immune Response.” *Nature Genetics* 50 (3): 424–31.

9. Alvarez, Mariano J., Yao Shen, Federico M. Giorgi, Alexander Lachmann, B. Belinda Ding, B. Hilda Ye, and Andrea Califano. 2016. "Functional Characterization of Somatic Mutations in Cancer Using Network-Based Inference of Protein Activity." *Nature Genetics* 48 (8): 838–47.

10. Aran, Dvir, Zicheng Hu, and Atul J. Butte. 2017. "XCell: Digitally Portraying the Tissue Cellular Heterogeneity Landscape." *Genome Biology* 18 (1): 220.

11. Arensbergen, Joris van, Ludo Pagie, Vincent D. FitzPatrick, Marcel de Haas, Marijke P. Baltissen, Federico Comoglio, Robin H. van der Weide, et al. 2019. "High-Throughput Identification of Human SNPs Affecting Regulatory Element Activity." *Nature Genetics* 51 (7): 1160–69.

12. Astle, William J., Heather Elding, Tao Jiang, Dave Allen, Dace Ruklisa, Alice L. Mann, Daniel Mead, et al. 2016. "The Allelic Landscape of Human Blood Cell Trait Variation and Links to Common Complex Disease." *Cell* 167 (5): 1415-1429.e19.

13. Baldán, Angel, Liming Pei, Richard Lee, Paul Tarr, Rajendra K. Tangirala, Michael M. Weinstein, Joy Frank, Andrew C. Li, Peter Tontonoz, and Peter A. Edwards. 2006. "Impaired Development of Atherosclerosis in Hyperlipidemic Ldlr-/- and ApoE-/- Mice Transplanted with Abcg1-/- Bone Marrow." *Arteriosclerosis, Thrombosis, and Vascular Biology* 26 (10): 2301–7.

14. Barbeira, Alvaro N., Rodrigo Bonazzola, Eric R. Gamazon, Yanyu Liang, Yoson Park, Sarah Kim-Hellmuth, Gao Wang, et al. 2021. "Exploiting the GTEx Resources to Decipher the Mechanisms at GWAS Loci." *Genome Biology* 22 (1): 49.

15. Barreiro, Luis B., Ludovic Tailleux, Athma A. Pai, Brigitte Gicquel, John C. Marioni, and Yoav Gilad. 2012. "Deciphering the Genetic Architecture of Variation in the Immune Response to Mycobacterium Tuberculosis Infection." *Proceedings of the National Academy of Sciences of the United States of America* 109 (4): 1204–9.

16. Barski, Artem, Suresh Cuddapah, Kairong Cui, Tae-Young Roh, Dustin E. Schones, Zhibin Wang, Gang Wei, Iouri Chepelev, and Keji Zhao. 2007. "High-Resolution Profiling of Histone Methylations in the Human Genome." *Cell* 129 (4): 823–37.

17. Benjamini, Yoav, and Yosef Hochberg. 1995. "Controlling the False Discovery Rate: A Practical and Powerful Approach to Multiple Testing." *Journal of the Royal Statistical Society. Series B, Statistical Methodology* 57 (1): 289–300.

18. Boyle, Alan P., Sean Davis, Hennady P. Shulha, Paul Meltzer, Elliott H. Margulies, Zhiping Weng, Terrence S. Furey, and Gregory E. Crawford. 2008. "High-Resolution Mapping and Characterization of Open Chromatin across the Genome." *Cell* 132 (2): 311–22.

19. Brandt, Margot, Alper Gokden, Marcello Ziosi, and Tuuli Lappalainen. 2020. "A Polyclonal Allelic Expression Assay for Detecting Regulatory Effects of Transcript Variants." *Genome Medicine* 12 (1): 79.

20. Brandt, Margot, Sarah Kim-Hellmuth, Marcello Ziosi, Alper Gokden, Aaron Wolman, Nora Lam, Yocelyn Recinos, Veit Hornung, Johannes Schumacher, and Tuuli Lappalainen. 2020. "An Autoimmune Disease Risk Variant Has a Trans Master Regulatory Effect Mediated by IRF1 under Immune Stimulation." *Cold Spring Harbor Laboratory*. https://doi.org/10.1101/2020.02.21.959734.

21. Brandt, Margot, and Tuuli Lappalainen. 2017. "SnapShot: Discovering Genetic Regulatory Variants by QTL Analysis." *Cell.*

22. Brasier, A. R., J. E. Tate, and J. F. Habener. 1989. "Optimized Use of the Firefly Luciferase Assay as a Reporter Gene in Mammalian Cell Lines." *BioTechniques* 7 (10): 1116–22.

23. Brown, Andrew Anand, Ana Viñuela, Olivier Delaneau, Tim D. Spector, Kerrin S. Small, and Emmanouil T. Dermitzakis. 2017. "Predicting Causal Variants Affecting Expression by Using Whole-Genome Sequencing and RNA-Seq from Multiple Human Tissues." *Nature Genetics* 49 (12): 1747–51.

24. Buenrostro, Jason D., Paul G. Giresi, Lisa C. Zaba, Howard Y. Chang, and William J. Greenleaf. 2013. "Transposition of Native Chromatin for Fast and Sensitive Epigenomic Profiling of Open Chromatin, DNA-Binding Proteins and Nucleosome Position." *Nature Methods* 10 (12): 1213–18.

25. Cano-Gamez, Eddie, and Gosia Trynka. 2020. "From GWAS to Function: Using Functional Genomics to Identify the Mechanisms Underlying Complex Diseases." *Frontiers in Genetics* 11 (May): 424.

26. CARDIoGRAMplusC4D Consortium, Panos Deloukas, Stavroula Kanoni, Christina Willenborg, Martin Farrall, Themistocles L. Assimes, John R. Thompson, et al. 2013. "Large-Scale Association Analysis Identifies New Risk Loci for Coronary Artery Disease." *Nature Genetics* 45 (1): 25–33.

27. Castel, Stephane E., Pejman Mohammadi, Wendy K. Chung, Yufeng Shen, and Tuuli Lappalainen. 2016. "Rare Variant Phasing and Haplotypic Expression from RNA Sequencing with PhASER." *Nature Communications* 7 (September): 12817.

28. CDC. 2021. "Coronary Artery Disease." July 19, 2021. https://www.cdc.gov/heartdisease/coronary_ad.htm.

29. Chandra, Vivek, Sourya Bhattacharyya, Benjamin J. Schmiedel, Ariel Madrigal, Cristian Gonzalez-Colin, Stephanie Fotsing, Austin Crinklaw, et al. 2021. "Promoter-Interacting

Expression Quantitative Trait Loci Are Enriched for Functional Genetic Variants." *Nature Genetics* 53 (1): 110–19.

30. Chang, Chieh, Carolyn E. Adler, Matthias Krause, Scott G. Clark, Frank B. Gertler, Marc Tessier-Lavigne, and Cornelia I. Bargmann. 2006. "MIG-10/Lamellipodin and AGE-1/PI3K Promote Axon Guidance and Outgrowth in Response to Slit and Netrin." *Current Biology: CB* 16 (9): 854–62.

31. Chen, Jieming, Joel Rozowsky, Timur R. Galeev, Arif Harmanci, Robert Kitchen, Jason Bedford, Alexej Abyzov, Yong Kong, Lynne Regan, and Mark Gerstein. 2016. "A Uniform Survey of Allele-Specific Binding and Expression over 1000-Genomes-Project Individuals." *Nature Communications* 7 (April): 11101.

32. Chen, Lu, Bing Ge, Francesco Paolo Casale, Louella Vasquez, Tony Kwan, Diego Garrido-Martín, Stephen Watt, et al. 2016. "Genetic Drivers of Epigenetic and Transcriptional Variation in Human Immune Cells." *Cell* 167 (5): 1398-1414.e24.

33. Chick, Joel M., Steven C. Munger, Petr Simecek, Edward L. Huttlin, Kwangbom Choi, Daniel M. Gatti, Narayanan Raghupathy, Karen L. Svenson, Gary A. Churchill, and Steven P. Gygi. 2016. "Defining the Consequences of Genetic Variation on a Proteome-Wide Scale." *Nature* 534 (7608): 500–505.

34. Chistiakov, Dimitry A., Yuri V. Bobryshev, and Alexander N. Orekhov. 2016. "Macrophage-Mediated Cholesterol Handling in Atherosclerosis." *Journal of Cellular and Molecular Medicine* 20 (1): 17–28.

35. Cooper, D. N., and M. Krawczak. 1996. "Human Gene Mutation Database." *Human Genetics* 98 (5): 629.

36. Coronary Artery Disease (C4D) Genetics Consortium. 2011. "A Genome-Wide Association Study in Europeans and South Asians Identifies Five New Loci for Coronary Artery Disease." *Nature Genetics* 43 (4): 339–44.

37. Cunningham, Fiona, Premanand Achuthan, Wasiu Akanni, James Allen, M. Ridwan Amode, Irina M. Armean, Ruth Bennett, et al. 2019. "Ensembl 2019." *Nucleic Acids Research* 47 (D1): D745–51.

38. Cuomo, Anna S. E., Daniel D. Seaton, Davis J. McCarthy, Iker Martinez, Marc Jan Bonder, Jose Garcia-Bernardo, Shradha Amatya, et al. 2020. "Single-Cell RNA-Sequencing of Differentiating IPS Cells Reveals Dynamic Genetic Effects on Gene Expression." *Nature Communications* 11 (1): 810.

39. Dai, Xiao-Yan, Yan Cai, Ding-Ding Mao, Yong-Fen Qi, Chaoshu Tang, Qingbo Xu, Yi Zhu, Ming-Jiang Xu, and Xian Wang. 2012. "Increased Stability of Phosphatase and Tensin Homolog by Intermedin Leading to Scavenger Receptor A Inhibition of

Macrophages Reduces Atherosclerosis in Apolipoprotein E-Deficient Mice." *Journal of Molecular and Cellular Cardiology* 53 (4): 509–20.

40. Davis, Joe R., Laure Frésard, David A. Knowles, Mauro Pala, Carlos D. Bustamante, Alexis Battle, and Stephen B. Montgomery. 2016. "An Efficient Multiple-Testing Adjustment for EQTL Studies That Accounts for Linkage Disequilibrium between Variants." *American Journal of Human Genetics* 98 (1): 216–24.

41. Degner, Jacob F., Athma A. Pai, Roger Pique-Regi, Jean-Baptiste Veyrieras, Daniel J. Gaffney, Joseph K. Pickrell, Sherryl De Leon, et al. 2012. "DNase I Sensitivity QTLs Are a Major Determinant of Human Expression Variation." *Nature* 482 (7385): 390–94.

42. DeKoter, R. P., J. C. Walsh, and H. Singh. 1998. "PU.1 Regulates Both Cytokine-Dependent Proliferation and Differentiation of Granulocyte/Macrophage Progenitors." *The EMBO Journal* 17 (15): 4456–68.

43. Ding, Zhihao, Yunyun Ni, Sander W. Timmer, Bum-Kyu Lee, Anna Battenhouse, Sandra Louzada, Fengtang Yang, et al. 2014. "Quantitative Genetics of CTCF Binding Reveal Local Sequence Effects and Different Modes of X-Chromosome Association." *PLoS Genetics* 10 (11): e1004798.

44. Dombroski, Beth A., Renuka R. Nayak, Kathryn G. Ewens, Wendy Ankener, Vivian G. Cheung, and Richard S. Spielman. 2010. "Gene Expression and Genetic Variation in Response to Endoplasmic Reticulum Stress in Human Cells." *American Journal of Human Genetics* 86 (5): 719–29.

45. EMBL-EBI. 2021. "The Ensembl Regulatory Build." Ensembl. May 1, 2021. http://may2021.archive.ensembl.org/info/genome/funcgen/regulatory_build.html.

46. ENCODE Project Consortium. 2012. "An Integrated Encyclopedia of DNA Elements in the Human Genome." *Nature* 489 (7414): 57–74.

47. ENCODE Project Consortium, Ewan Birney, John A. Stamatoyannopoulos, Anindya Dutta, Roderic Guigó, Thomas R. Gingeras, Elliott H. Margulies, et al. 2007. "Identification and Analysis of Functional Elements in 1% of the Human Genome by the ENCODE Pilot Project." *Nature* 447 (7146): 799–816.

48. Evans, Trent D., Xiangyu Zhang, Reece E. Clark, Arturo Alisio, Eric Song, Hanrui Zhang, Muredach P. Reilly, Nathan O. Stitziel, and Babak Razani. 2019. "Functional Characterization of LIPA (Lysosomal Acid Lipase) Variants Associated With Coronary Artery Disease." *Arteriosclerosis, Thrombosis, and Vascular Biology* 39 (12): 2480–91.

49. Ezzat, Shereen, Rene Mader, Sandra Fischer, Shunjiang Yu, Cameron Ackerley, and Sylvia L. Asa. 2006. "An Essential Role for the Hematopoietic Transcription Factor

Ikaros in Hypothalamic-Pituitary-Mediated Somatic Growth." *Proceedings of the National Academy of Sciences of the United States of America* 103 (7): 2214–19.

50. Fairfax, Benjamin P., Peter Humburg, Seiko Makino, Vivek Naranbhai, Daniel Wong, Evelyn Lau, Luke Jostins, et al. 2014. "Innate Immune Activity Conditions the Effect of Regulatory Variants upon Monocyte Gene Expression." *Science* 343 (6175): 1246949.

51. Fairfax, Benjamin P., Seiko Makino, Jayachandran Radhakrishnan, Katharine Plant, Stephen Leslie, Alexander Dilthey, Peter Ellis, Cordelia Langford, Fredrik O. Vannberg, and Julian C. Knight. 2012. "Genetics of Gene Expression in Primary Immune Cells Identifies Cell Type-Specific Master Regulators and Roles of HLA Alleles." *Nature Genetics* 44 (5): 502–10.

52. Fazio, S., A. S. Major, L. L. Swift, L. A. Gleaves, M. Accad, M. F. Linton, and R. V. Farese Jr. 2001. "Increased Atherosclerosis in LDL Receptor-Null Mice Lacking ACAT1 in Macrophages." *The Journal of Clinical Investigation* 107 (2): 163–71.

53. Findley, Anthony S., Alan Monziani, Allison L. Richards, Katherine Rhodes, Michelle C. Ward, Cynthia A. Kalita, Adnan Alazizi, et al. 2021. "Functional Dynamic Genetic Effects on Gene Regulation Are Specific to Particular Cell Types and Environmental Conditions." *ELife* 10 (May). https://doi.org/10.7554/eLife.67077.

54. Findley, Anthony S., Allison L. Richards, Cristiano Petrini, Adnan Alazizi, Elizabeth Doman, Alexander G. Shanku, Gordon O. Davis, et al. 2019. "Interpreting Coronary Artery Disease Risk Through Gene-Environment Interactions in Gene Regulation." *Genetics*, September, genetics.302419.2019-12.

55. Flynn, Elise, Athena L. Tsu, Silva Kasela, Sarah Kim-Hellmuth, Francois Aguet, Kristin G. Ardlie, Harmen J. Bussemaker, Pejman Mohammadi, and Tuuli Lappalainen. 2021. "Transcription Factor Regulation of EQTL Activity across Individuals and Tissues." *BioRxiv*. https://doi.org/10.1101/2021.07.20.453075.

56. Gaffney, Daniel J., Jean-Baptiste Veyrieras, Jacob F. Degner, Roger Pique-Regi, Athma A. Pai, Gregory E. Crawford, Matthew Stephens, Yoav Gilad, and Jonathan K. Pritchard. 2012. "Dissecting the Regulatory Architecture of Gene Expression QTLs." *Genome Biology* 13 (1): R7.

57. Gao, Xiaoyi, Joshua Starmer, and Eden R. Martin. 2008. "A Multiple Testing Correction Method for Genetic Association Studies Using Correlated Single Nucleotide Polymorphisms." *Genetic Epidemiology* 32 (4): 361–69.

58. Garcia-Alonso, Luz, Christian H. Holland, Mahmoud M. Ibrahim, Denes Turei, and Julio Saez-Rodriguez. 2019. "Benchmark and Integration of Resources for the Estimation of Human Transcription Factor Activities." *Genome Research* 29 (8): 1363–75.

59. Garieri, Marco, Olivier Delaneau, Federico Santoni, Richard J. Fish, David Mull, Piero Carninci, Emmanouil T. Dermitzakis, Stylianos E. Antonarakis, and Alexandre Fort. 2017. "The Effect of Genetic Variation on Promoter Usage and Enhancer Activity." *Nature Communications* 8 (1): 1358.

60. Garner, M. M., and A. Revzin. 1981. "A Gel Electrophoresis Method for Quantifying the Binding of Proteins to Specific DNA Regions: Application to Components of the Escherichia Coli Lactose Operon Regulatory System." *Nucleic Acids Research* 9 (13): 3047–60.

61. Geijn, Bryce van de, Graham McVicker, Yoav Gilad, and Jonathan K. Pritchard. 2015. "WASP: Allele-Specific Software for Robust Molecular Quantitative Trait Locus Discovery." *Nature Methods* 12 (11): 1061–63.

62. Georgopoulos, Katia. 2002. "Haematopoietic Cell-Fate Decisions, Chromatin Regulation and Ikaros." *Nature Reviews. Immunology* 2 (3): 162–74.

63. Giambartolomei, Claudia, Damjan Vukcevic, Eric E. Schadt, Lude Franke, Aroon D. Hingorani, Chris Wallace, and Vincent Plagnol. 2014. "Bayesian Test for Colocalisation between Pairs of Genetic Association Studies Using Summary Statistics." *PLoS Genetics* 10 (5): e1004383-15.

64. Glinos, Dafni A., Garrett Garborcauskas, Paul Hoffman, Nava Ehsan, Lihua Jiang, Alper Gokden, Xiaoguang Dai, et al. 2021. "Transcriptome Variation in Human Tissues Revealed by Long-Read Sequencing." *BioRxiv*. https://doi.org/10.1101/2021.01.22.427687.

65. Greenbaum, Dov, Christopher Colangelo, Kenneth Williams, and Mark Gerstein. 2003. "Comparing Protein Abundance and MRNA Expression Levels on a Genomic Scale." *Genome Biology* 4 (9): 117.

66. Gregoire, F. M., C. M. Smas, and H. S. Sul. 1998. "Understanding Adipocyte Differentiation." *Physiological Reviews* 78 (3): 783–809.

67. Grubert, Fabian, Judith B. Zaugg, Maya Kasowski, Oana Ursu, Damek V. Spacek, Alicia R. Martin, Peyton Greenside, et al. 2015. "Genetic Control of Chromatin States in Humans Involves Local and Distal Chromosomal Interactions." *Cell* 162 (5): 1051–65.

68. Gry, Marcus, Rebecca Rimini, Sara Strömberg, Anna Asplund, Fredrik Pontén, Mathias Uhlén, and Peter Nilsson. 2009. "Correlations between RNA and Protein Expression Profiles in 23 Human Cell Lines." *BMC Genomics* 10 (August): 365.

69. GTEx Consortium. 2015. "The Genotype-Tissue Expression (GTEx) Pilot Analysis: Multitissue Gene Regulation in Humans." *Science* 348 (6235): 648–60.

70. ———. 2020. "The GTEx Consortium Atlas of Genetic Regulatory Effects across Human Tissues." *Science* 369 (6509): 1318–30.

71. GTEx Consortium, François Aguet, Andrew Anand Brown, Stephane E. Castel, Joe R. Davis, Yuan He, Brian Jo, et al. 2017. "Genetic Effects on Gene Expression across Human Tissues." *Nature Publishing Group* 550 (7675): 204–13.

72. Gupta, Rajat M., Joseph Hadaya, Aditi Trehan, Seyedeh M. Zekavat, Carolina Roselli, Derek Klarin, Connor A. Emdin, et al. 2017. "A Genetic Variant Associated with Five Vascular Diseases Is a Distal Regulator of Endothelin-1 Gene Expression." *Cell* 170 (3): 522-533.e15.

73. Gutierrez-Arcelus, Maria, Yuriy Baglaenko, Jatin Arora, Susan Hannes, Yang Luo, Tiffany Amariuta, Nikola Teslovich, et al. 2020. "Allele-Specific Expression Changes Dynamically during T Cell Activation in HLA and Other Autoimmune Loci." *Nature Genetics*, February, 1–23.

74. Gutierrez-Arcelus, Maria, Halit Ongen, Tuuli Lappalainen, Stephen B. Montgomery, Alfonso Buil, Alisa Yurovsky, Julien Bryois, et al. 2015. "Tissue-Specific Effects of Genetic and Epigenetic Variation on Gene Regulation and Splicing." *PLoS Genetics* 11 (1): e1004958.

75. Handberg, A., K. Højlund, A. Gastaldelli, A. Flyvbjerg, J. M. Dekker, J. Petrie, P. Piatti, H. Beck-Nielsen, and RISC Investigators. 2012. "Plasma SCD36 Is Associated with Markers of Atherosclerosis, Insulin Resistance and Fatty Liver in a Nondiabetic Healthy Population." *Journal of Internal Medicine* 271 (3): 294–304.

76. Harst, Pim van der, and Niek Verweij. 2018. "Identification of 64 Novel Genetic Loci Provides an Expanded View on the Genetic Architecture of Coronary Artery Disease." *Circulation Research* 122 (3): 433–43.

77. Hayden, Matthew S., and Sankar Ghosh. 2011. "NF-KB in Immunobiology." *Cell Research* 21 (2): 223–44.

78. He, Bing, Jian Shi, Xinwen Wang, Hui Jiang, and Hao-Jie Zhu. 2020. "Genome-Wide PQTL Analysis of Protein Expression Regulatory Networks in the Human Liver." *BMC Biology* 18 (1): 97.

79. He, Yuan, Surya B. Chhetri, Marios Arvanitis, Kaushik Srinivasan, François Aguet, Kristin G. Ardlie, Alvaro N. Barbeira, et al. 2020. "Sn-SpMF: Matrix Factorization Informs Tissue-Specific Genetic Regulation of Gene Expression." *Genome Biology* 21 (1): 235.

80. Heintzman, Nathaniel D., Gary C. Hon, R. David Hawkins, Pouya Kheradpour, Alexander Stark, Lindsey F. Harp, Zhen Ye, et al. 2009. "Histone Modifications at

Human Enhancers Reflect Global Cell-Type-Specific Gene Expression." *Nature* 459 (7243): 108–12.

81. Heinzen, Erin L., Dongliang Ge, Kenneth D. Cronin, Jessica M. Maia, Kevin V. Shianna, Willow N. Gabriel, Kathleen A. Welsh-Bohmer, Christine M. Hulette, Thomas N. Denny, and David B. Goldstein. 2008. "Tissue-Specific Genetic Control of Splicing: Implications for the Study of Complex Traits." *PLoS Biology* 6 (12): e1.

82. Hillmer, Emily J., Huiyuan Zhang, Haiyan S. Li, and Stephanie S. Watowich. 2016. "STAT3 Signaling in Immunity." *Cytokine & Growth Factor Reviews* 31 (October): 1–15.

83. Hormozdiari, Farhad, Martijn van de Bunt, Ayellet V. Segre, Xiao Li, Jong Wha J. Joo, Michael Bilow, Jae Hoon Sul, Sriram Sankararaman, Bogdan Pasaniuc, and Eleazar Eskin. 2016. "Colocalization of GWAS and EQTL Signals Detects Target Genes." *American Journal of Human Genetics* 99 (6): 1245–60.

84. Hormozdiari, Farhad, Emrah Kostem, Eun Yong Kang, Bogdan Pasaniuc, and Eleazar Eskin. 2014. "Identifying Causal Variants at Loci with Multiple Signals of Association." *Genetics*, October, 1–21.

85. Hu Frisk, Jun Mei, Lena Kjellén, Stephen G. Kaler, Gunnar Pejler, and Helena Öhrvik. 2017. "Copper Regulates Maturation and Expression of an MITF:Tryptase Axis in Mast Cells." *Journal of Immunology* 199 (12): 4132–41.

86. IBC 50K CAD Consortium. 2011. "Large-Scale Gene-Centric Analysis Identifies Novel Variants for Coronary Artery Disease." *PLoS Genetics* 7 (9): e1002260.

87. Igarashi, Masaki, Jun-Ichi Osuga, Hiroshi Uozaki, Motohiro Sekiya, Shuichi Nagashima, Manabu Takahashi, Satoru Takase, et al. 2010. "The Critical Role of Neutral Cholesterol Ester Hydrolase 1 in Cholesterol Removal from Human Macrophages." *Circulation Research* 107 (11): 1387–95.

88. Inoue, Fumitaka, Martin Kircher, Beth Martin, Gregory M. Cooper, Daniela M. Witten, Michael T. McManus, Nadav Ahituv, and Jay Shendure. 2017. "A Systematic Comparison Reveals Substantial Differences in Chromosomal versus Episomal Encoding of Enhancer Activity." *Genome Research* 27 (1): 38–52.

89. Irvine, W. J., F. C. W. Wu, S. J. Urbaniak, and F. TOOLIS Endocrinology and. 1977. "Peripheral Blood Leucocytes in Thyrotoxicosis." *Clinical and Experimental Immunology* 27: 216–21.

90. Jerber, Julie, Daniel D. Seaton, Anna S. E. Cuomo, Natsuhiko Kumasaka, James Haldane, Juliette Steer, Minal Patel, et al. 2021. "Population-Scale Single-Cell RNA-Seq Profiling across Dopaminergic Neuron Differentiation." *Nature Genetics* 53 (3): 304–12.

91. Jiang, Lihua, Meng Wang, Shin Lin, Ruiqi Jian, Xiao Li, Joanne Chan, Guanlan Dong, et al. 2020. "A Quantitative Proteome Map of the Human Body." *Cell* 183 (1): 269-283.e19.

92. Jinek, Martin, Krzysztof Chylinski, Ines Fonfara, Michael Hauer, Jennifer A. Doudna, and Emmanuelle Charpentier. 2012. "A Programmable Dual-RNA-Guided DNA Endonuclease in Adaptive Bacterial Immunity." *Science* 337 (6096): 816–21.

93. Johnson, David S., Ali Mortazavi, Richard M. Myers, and Barbara Wold. 2007. "Genome-Wide Mapping of in Vivo Protein-DNA Interactions." *Science* 316 (5830): 1497–1502.

94. Jolma, Arttu, Teemu Kivioja, Jarkko Toivonen, Lu Cheng, Gonghong Wei, Martin Enge, Mikko Taipale, et al. 2010. "Multiplexed Massively Parallel SELEX for Characterization of Human Transcription Factor Binding Specificities." *Genome Research* 20 (6): 861–73.

95. Jolma, Arttu, Jian Yan, Thomas Whitington, Jarkko Toivonen, Kazuhiro R. Nitta, Pasi Rastas, Ekaterina Morgunova, et al. 2013. "DNA-Binding Specificities of Human Transcription Factors." *Cell* 152 (1–2): 327–39.

96. Kariuki, Silvia N., Joseph C. Maranville, Shaneen S. Baxter, Choongwon Jeong, Shigeki Nakagome, Cara L. Hrusch, David B. Witonsky, Anne I. Sperling, and Anna Di Rienzo. 2016. "Mapping Variation in Cellular and Transcriptional Response to 1,25-Dihydroxyvitamin D3 in Peripheral Blood Mononuclear Cells." *PloS One* 11 (7): e0159779.

97. Kasela, Silva, Kai Kisand, Liina Tserel, Epp Kaleviste, Anu Remm, Krista Fischer, Tõnu Esko, et al. 2017. "Pathogenic Implications for Autoimmune Mechanisms Derived by Comparative EQTL Analysis of CD4+ versus CD8+ T Cells." *PLoS Genetics* 13 (3): e1006643.

98. Kasowski, Maya, Sofia Kyriazopoulou-Panagiotopoulou, Fabian Grubert, Judith B. Zaugg, Anshul Kundaje, Yuling Liu, Alan P. Boyle, et al. 2013. "Extensive Variation in Chromatin States across Humans." *Science* 342 (6159): 750–52.

99. Kelley, David R., Jasper Snoek, and John L. Rinn. 2016. "Basset: Learning the Regulatory Code of the Accessible Genome with Deep Convolutional Neural Networks." *Genome Research* 26 (7): 990–99.

100. Kerem, B., J. M. Rommens, J. A. Buchanan, D. Markiewicz, T. K. Cox, A. Chakravarti, M. Buchwald, and L. C. Tsui. 1989. "Identification of the Cystic Fibrosis Gene: Genetic Analysis." *Science* 245 (4922): 1073–80.

101. Kheradpour, Pouya, Jason Ernst, Alexandre Melnikov, Peter Rogov, Li Wang, Xiaolan Zhang, Jessica Alston, Tarjei S. Mikkelsen, and Manolis Kellis. 2013. "Systematic

Dissection of Regulatory Motifs in 2000 Predicted Human Enhancers Using a Massively Parallel Reporter Assay." *Genome Research* 23 (5): 800–811.

102. Kheradpour, Pouya, and Manolis Kellis. 2014. "Systematic Discovery and Characterization of Regulatory Motifs in ENCODE TF Binding Experiments." *Nucleic Acids Research* 42 (5): 2976–87.

103. Kichaev, Gleb, Gaurav Bhatia, Po-Ru Loh, Steven Gazal, Kathryn Burch, Malika K. Freund, Armin Schoech, Bogdan Pasaniuc, and Alkes L. Price. 2019. "Leveraging Polygenic Functional Enrichment to Improve GWAS Power." *American Journal of Human Genetics* 104 (1): 65–75.

104. Kichaev, Gleb, Wen-Yun Yang, Sara Lindstrom, Farhad Hormozdiari, Eleazar Eskin, Alkes L. Price, Peter Kraft, and Bogdan Pasaniuc. 2014. "Integrating Functional Data to Prioritize Causal Variants in Statistical Fine-Mapping Studies." *PLoS Genetics* 10 (10): e1004722-16.

105. Kilpinen, Helena, Sebastian M. Waszak, Andreas R. Gschwind, Sunil K. Raghav, Robert M. Witwicki, Andrea Orioli, Eugenia Migliavacca, et al. 2013. "Coordinated Effects of Sequence Variation on DNA Binding, Chromatin Structure, and Transcription." *Science*, November, 1–5.

106. Kim, Sarah, Jessica Becker, Matthias Bechheim, Vera Kaiser, Mahdad Noursadeghi, Nadine Fricker, Esther Beier, et al. 2014. "Characterizing the Genetic Basis of Innate Immune Response in TLR4-Activated Human Monocytes." *Nature Communications* 5 (October): 5236.

107. Kim-Hellmuth, Sarah, François Aguet, Meritxell Oliva, Manuel Muñoz-Aguirre, Silva Kasela, Valentin Wucher, Stephane E. Castel, et al. 2020. "Cell Type-Specific Genetic Regulation of Gene Expression across Human Tissues." *Science* 369 (6509). https://doi.org/10.1126/science.aaz8528.

108. Kim-Hellmuth, Sarah, Matthias Bechheim, Benno Pütz, Pejman Mohammadi, Yohann Nédélec, Nicholas Giangreco, Jessica Becker, et al. 2017. "Genetic Regulatory Effects Modified by Immune Activation Contribute to Autoimmune Disease Associations." *Nature Communications*, August, 1–10.

109. Kimura, Kouichi, Ai Wakamatsu, Yutaka Suzuki, Toshio Ota, Tetsuo Nishikawa, Riu Yamashita, Jun-Ichi Yamamoto, et al. 2006. "Diversification of Transcriptional Modulation: Large-Scale Identification and Characterization of Putative Alternative Promoters of Human Genes." *Genome Research* 16 (1): 55–65.

110. Knowles, David A., Courtney K. Burrows, John D. Blischak, Kristen M. Patterson, Daniel J. Serie, Nadine Norton, Carole Ober, Jonathan K. Pritchard, and Yoav Gilad. 2018. "Determining the Genetic Basis of Anthracycline-Cardiotoxicity by Molecular

Response QTL Mapping in Induced Cardiomyocytes." *ELife* 7 (May). https://doi.org/10.7554/eLife.33480.

111. Knowles, David A., Joe R. Davis, Hilary Edgington, Anil Raj, Marie-Julie Favé, Xiaowei Zhu, James B. Potash, et al. 2017. "Allele-Specific Expression Reveals Interactions between Genetic Variation and Environment." *Nature Publishing Group*, May, 1–6.

112. Koyama, Satoshi, Kaoru Ito, Chikashi Terao, Masato Akiyama, Momoko Horikoshi, Yukihide Momozawa, Hiroshi Matsunaga, et al. 2020. "Population-Specific and Trans-Ancestry Genome-Wide Analyses Identify Distinct and Shared Genetic Risk Loci for Coronary Artery Disease." *Nature Genetics* 52 (11): 1169–77.

113. Kubota, Naoto, and Mikita Suyama. 2021. "Functional Variants in Hematopoietic Transcription Factor Footprints and Their Roles in the Risk of Immune System Diseases." *BioRxiv*. https://doi.org/10.1101/2021.03.22.436360.

114. Kulakovskiy, Ivan V., Ilya E. Vorontsov, Ivan S. Yevshin, Ruslan N. Sharipov, Alla D. Fedorova, Eugene I. Rumynskiy, Yulia A. Medvedeva, et al. 2018. "HOCOMOCO: Towards a Complete Collection of Transcription Factor Binding Models for Human and Mouse via Large-Scale ChIP-Seq Analysis." *Nucleic Acids Research* 46 (D1): D252–59.

115. Kurosaki, Tatsuaki, Maximilian W. Popp, and Lynne E. Maquat. 2019. "Quality and Quantity Control of Gene Expression by Nonsense-Mediated MRNA Decay." *Nature Reviews. Molecular Cell Biology* 20 (7): 406–20.

116. Lafuente, Esther M., André A. F. L. van Puijenbroek, Matthias Krause, Christopher V. Carman, Gordon J. Freeman, Alla Berezovskaya, Erica Constantine, Timothy A. Springer, Frank B. Gertler, and Vassiliki A. Boussiotis. 2004. "RIAM, an Ena/VASP and Profilin Ligand, Interacts with Rap1-GTP and Mediates Rap1-Induced Adhesion." *Developmental Cell* 7 (4): 585–95.

117. Lagarrigue, Frederic, Chungho Kim, and Mark H. Ginsberg. 2016. "The Rap1-RIAM-Talin Axis of Integrin Activation and Blood Cell Function." *Blood* 128 (4): 479–87.

118. Lagarrigue, Frederic, Praju Vikas Anekal, Ho-Sup Lee, Alexia I. Bachir, Jailal N. Ablack, Alan F. Horwitz, and Mark H. Ginsberg. 2015. "A RIAM/Lamellipodin-Talin-Integrin Complex Forms the Tip of Sticky Fingers That Guide Cell Migration." *Nature Communications* 6 (September): 8492.

119. Landrum, Melissa J., Jennifer M. Lee, George R. Riley, Wonhee Jang, Wendy S. Rubinstein, Deanna M. Church, and Donna R. Maglott. 2014. "ClinVar: Public Archive of Relationships among Sequence Variation and Human Phenotype." *Nucleic Acids Research* 42 (Database issue): D980-5.

120. Lappalainen, Tuuli, Michael Sammeth, Marc R. Friedländer, Peter A. C. 't Hoen, Jean Monlong, Manuel A. Rivas, Mar Gonzàlez-Porta, et al. 2013. "Transcriptome and Genome Sequencing Uncovers Functional Variation in Humans." *Nature* 501 (7468): 506–11.

121. Leblanc, Benoît, and Tom Moss, eds. 2009. *DNA-Protein Interactions: Principles and Protocols, Third Edition*. Humana Press.

122. Lee, Mark N., Chun Ye, Alexandra-Chloé Villani, Towfique Raj, Weibo Li, Thomas M. Eisenhaure, Selina H. Imboywa, et al. 2014. "Common Genetic Variants Modulate Pathogen-Sensing Responses in Human Dendritic Cells." *Science* 343 (6175): 1246980.

123. Lee, Yeji, Francesca Luca, Roger Pique-Regi, and Xiaoquan Wen. 2018. "Bayesian Multi-SNP Genetic Association Analysis: Control of FDR and Use of Summary Statistics." *BioRxiv*. https://doi.org/10.1101/316471.

124. Lin, Yao-Cheng, Morgane Boone, Leander Meuris, Irma Lemmens, Nadine Van Roy, Arne Soete, Joke Reumers, et al. 2014. "Genome Dynamics of the Human Embryonic Kidney 293 Lineage in Response to Cell Biology Manipulations." *Nature Communications* 5 (September): 4767.

125. López-Martínez, Andrea, Patricia Soblechero-Martín, Laura de-la-Puente-Ovejero, Gisela Nogales-Gadea, and Virginia Arechavala-Gomeza. 2020. "An Overview of Alternative Splicing Defects Implicated in Myotonic Dystrophy Type I." *Genes* 11 (9). https://doi.org/10.3390/genes11091109.

126. Lou, Hong, Meredith Yeager, Hongchuan Li, Jesus Gonzalez Bosquet, Richard B. Hayes, Nick Orr, Kai Yu, et al. 2009. "Fine Mapping and Functional Analysis of a Common Variant in MSMB on Chromosome 10q11.2 Associated with Prostate Cancer Susceptibility." *Proceedings of the National Academy of Sciences of the United States of America* 106 (19): 7933–38.

127. Love, Michael I., Wolfgang Huber, and Simon Anders. 2014. "Moderated Estimation of Fold Change and Dispersion for RNA-Seq Data with DESeq2." *Genome Biology* 15 (12): 550.

128. Lukacs, Gergely L., and A. S. Verkman. 2012. "CFTR: Folding, Misfolding and Correcting the ΔF508 Conformational Defect." *Trends in Molecular Medicine* 18 (2): 81–91.

129. Mandric, Igor, Tommer Schwarz, Arunabha Majumdar, Kangcheng Hou, Leah Briscoe, Richard Perez, Meena Subramaniam, et al. 2020. "Optimized Design of Single-Cell RNA Sequencing Experiments for Cell-Type-Specific EQTL Analysis." *Nature Communications* 11 (1): 5504.

130. Maranville, Joseph C., Francesca Luca, Allison L. Richards, Xiaoquan Wen, David B. Witonsky, Shaneen Baxter, Matthew Stephens, and Anna Di Rienzo. 2011. "Interactions between Glucocorticoid Treatment and Cis-Regulatory Polymorphisms Contribute to Cellular Response Phenotypes." *PLoS Genetics* 7 (7): e1002162.

131. Mathelier, Anthony, Oriol Fornes, David J. Arenillas, Chih-Yu Chen, Grégoire Denay, Jessica Lee, Wenqiang Shi, et al. 2016. "JASPAR 2016: A Major Expansion and Update of the Open-Access Database of Transcription Factor Binding Profiles." *Nucleic Acids Research* 44 (D1): D110-5.

132. Matsunaga, Hiroshi, Kaoru Ito, Masato Akiyama, Atsushi Takahashi, Satoshi Koyama, Seitaro Nomura, Hirotaka Ieki, et al. 2020. "Transethnic Meta-Analysis of Genome-Wide Association Studies Identifies Three New Loci and Characterizes Population-Specific Differences for Coronary Artery Disease." *Circulation. Genomic and Precision Medicine* 13 (3): e002670.

133. McElwee, Matthew K., Min Ok Song, and Jonathan H. Freedman. 2009. "Copper Activation of NF-KappaB Signaling in HepG2 Cells." *Journal of Molecular Biology* 393 (5): 1013–21.

134. McLaren, William, Laurent Gil, Sarah E. Hunt, Harpreet Singh Riat, Graham R. S. Ritchie, Anja Thormann, Paul Flicek, and Fiona Cunningham. 2016. "The Ensembl Variant Effect Predictor." *Genome Biology* 17 (1): 122.

135. McVicker, Graham, Bryce van de Geijn, Jacob F. Degner, Carolyn E. Cain, Nicholas E. Banovich, Anil Raj, Noah Lewellen, Marsha Myrthil, Yoav Gilad, and Jonathan K. Pritchard. 2013. "Identification of Genetic Variants That Affect Histone Modifications in Human Cells." *Science* 342 (6159): 747–49.

136. Melnikov, Alexandre, Anand Murugan, Xiaolan Zhang, Tiberiu Tesileanu, Li Wang, Peter Rogov, Soheil Feizi, et al. 2012. "Systematic Dissection and Optimization of Inducible Enhancers in Human Cells Using a Massively Parallel Reporter Assay." *Nature Biotechnology* 30 (3): 271–77.

137. Meyer, Kerstin B., Martin O'Reilly, Kyriaki Michailidou, Saskia Carlebur, Stacey L. Edwards, Juliet D. French, Radhika Prathalingham, et al. 2013. "Fine-Scale Mapping of the FGFR2 Breast Cancer Risk Locus: Putative Functional Variants Differentially Bind FOXA1 and E2F1." *American Journal of Human Genetics* 93 (6): 1046–60.

138. Mirauta, Bogdan Andrei, Daniel D. Seaton, Dalila Bensaddek, Alejandro Brenes, Marc Jan Bonder, Helena Kilpinen, HipSci Consortium, Oliver Stegle, and Angus I. Lamond. 2020. "Population-Scale Proteome Variation in Human Induced Pluripotent Stem Cells." *ELife* 9 (August). https://doi.org/10.7554/eLife.57390.

139. Mizuno, Akira, and Yukinori Okada. 2019. "Biological Characterization of Expression Quantitative Trait Loci (EQTLs) Showing Tissue-Specific Opposite Directional Effects." *European Journal of Human Genetics: EJHG* 27 (11): 1745–56.

140. Mohammadi, Pejman, Stephane E. Castel, Andrew Anand Brown, and Tuuli Lappalainen. 2017a. "Quantifying the Regulatory Effect Size of Cis-Acting Genetic Variation Using Allelic Fold Change." *Genome Research* 27 (11): 1872–84.

141. ———. 2017b. "Quantifying the Regulatory Effect Size of Cis-Acting Genetic Variation Using Allelic Fold Change." *Genome Research* 27 (11): 1872–84.

142. Monlong, Jean, Miquel Calvo, Pedro G. Ferreira, and Roderic Guigó. 2014. "Identification of Genetic Variants Associated with Alternative Splicing Using SQTLseekeR." *Nature Communications* 5 (August): 4698.

143. Mouri, Kousuke, Michael H. Guo, Carl G. de Boer, Gregory A. Newby, Matteo Gentili, David R. Liu, Nir Hacohen, Ryan Tewhey, and John P. Ray. 2021. "Prioritization of Autoimmune Disease-Associated Genetic Variants That Perturb Regulatory Element Activity in T Cells." *BioRxiv*. https://doi.org/10.1101/2021.05.30.445673.

144. Moyerbrailean, Gregory A., Allison L. Richards, Daniel Kurtz, Cynthia A. Kalita, Gordon O. Davis, Chris T. Harvey, Adnan Alazizi, et al. 2016. "High-Throughput Allele-Specific Expression across 250 Environmental Conditions." *Genome Research* 26 (12): 1627–38.

145. Naranbhai, Vivek, Benjamin P. Fairfax, Seiko Makino, Peter Humburg, Daniel Wong, Esther Ng, Adrian V. S. Hill, and Julian C. Knight. 2015. "Genomic Modulators of Gene Expression in Human Neutrophils." *Nature Communications* 6 (July): 7545.

146. Neavin, Drew, Quan Nguyen, Maciej S. Daniszewski, Helena H. Liang, Han Sheng Chiu, Yong Kiat Wee, Anne Senabouth, et al. 2021. "Single Cell EQTL Analysis Identifies Cell Type-Specific Genetic Control of Gene Expression in Fibroblasts and Reprogrammed Induced Pluripotent Stem Cells." *Genome Biology* 22 (1): 76.

147. Nédélec, Yohann, Joaquín Sanz, Golshid Baharian, Zachary A. Szpiech, Alain Pacis, Anne Dumaine, Jean-Christophe Grenier, et al. 2016. "Genetic Ancestry and Natural Selection Drive Population Differences in Immune Responses to Pathogens." *Cell* 167 (3): 657-669.e21.

148. Nelson, Christopher P., Anuj Goel, Adam S. Butterworth, Stavroula Kanoni, Tom R. Webb, Eirini Marouli, Lingyao Zeng, et al. 2017. "Association Analyses Based on False Discovery Rate Implicate New Loci for Coronary Artery Disease." *Nature Genetics* 49 (9): 1385–91.

149. Ng, P. C., and S. Henikoff. 2001. "Predicting Deleterious Amino Acid Substitutions." *Genome Research* 11 (5): 863–74.

150. Nikpay, Majid, Anuj Goel, Hong-Hee Won, Leanne M. Hall, Christina Willenborg, Stavroula Kanoni, Danish Saleheen, et al. 2015. "A Comprehensive 1,000 Genomes-Based Genome-Wide Association Meta-Analysis of Coronary Artery Disease." *Nature Genetics* 47 (10): 1121–30.

151. Nikpay, Majid, Adam W. Turner, and Ruth McPherson. 2018. "Partitioning the Pleiotropy Between Coronary Artery Disease and Body Mass Index Reveals the Importance of Low Frequency Variants and Central Nervous System-Specific Functional Elements." *Circulation. Genomic and Precision Medicine* 11 (2): e002050.

152. Oh, Ji Hee, Young Jin Kim, Sanghoon Moon, Hye-Young Nam, Jae-Pil Jeon, Jong Ho Lee, Jong-Young Lee, and Yoon Shin Cho. 2013. "Genotype Instability during Long-Term Subculture of Lymphoblastoid Cell Lines." *Journal of Human Genetics* 58 (1): 16–20.

153. "OMIM - Online Mendelian Inheritance in Man." 1985. 1985. http://www.omim.org.

154. Ongen, Halit, Alfonso Buil, Emmanouil T. Dermitzakis, Olivier Delaneau, and Andrew Anand Brown. 2016. "Fast and Efficient QTL Mapper for Thousands of Molecular Phenotypes." *Bioinformatics* 32 (10): 1479–85.

155. Ortiga-Carvalho, Tânia M., Aniket R. Sidhaye, and Fredric E. Wondisford. 2014. "Thyroid Hormone Receptors and Resistance to Thyroid Hormone Disorders." *Nature Reviews. Endocrinology* 10 (10): 582–91.

156. Park, Yongjin, Liang He, Jose Davila-Velderrain, Lei Hou, Shahin Mohammadi, Hansruedi Mathys, Zhuyu Peng, David Bennett, Li-Huei Tsai, and Manolis Kellis. 2021. "Single-Cell Deconvolution of 3,000 Post-Mortem Brain Samples for EQTL and GWAS Dissection in Mental Disorders." *BioRxiv*. https://doi.org/10.1101/2021.01.21.426000.

157. Patel, Devanshi, Xiaoling Zhang, John J. Farrell, Jaeyoon Chung, Thor D. Stein, Kathryn L. Lunetta, and Lindsay A. Farrer. 2021. "Cell-Type-Specific Expression Quantitative Trait Loci Associated with Alzheimer Disease in Blood and Brain Tissue." *Translational Psychiatry* 11 (1): 250.

158. Patsoukis, Nikolaos, Kankana Bardhan, Jessica D. Weaver, Duygu Sari, Alvaro Torres-Gomez, Lequn Li, Laura Strauss, Esther M. Lafuente, and Vassiliki A. Boussiotis. 2017. "The Adaptor Molecule RIAM Integrates Signaling Events Critical for Integrin-Mediated Control of Immune Function and Cancer Progression." *Science Signaling* 10 (493). https://doi.org/10.1126/scisignal.aam8298.

159. PsychENCODE Consortium. 2018. "Revealing the Brain's Molecular Architecture." *Science* 362 (6420): 1262–63.

160. Raj, Towfique, Katie Rothamel, Sara Mostafavi, Chun Ye, Mark N. Lee, Joseph M. Replogle, Ting Feng, et al. 2014. "Polarization of the Effects of Autoimmune and Neurodegenerative Risk Alleles in Leukocytes." *Science* 344 (6183): 519–23.

161. Ran, F. Ann, Patrick D. Hsu, Jason Wright, Vineeta Agarwala, David A. Scott, and Feng Zhang. 2013. "Genome Engineering Using the CRISPR-Cas9 System." *Nature Protocols* 8 (11): 2281–2308.

162. Ranalletta, Mollie, Nan Wang, Seongah Han, Laurent Yvan-Charvet, Carrie Welch, and Alan R. Tall. 2006. "Decreased Atherosclerosis in Low-Density Lipoprotein Receptor Knockout Mice Transplanted with Abcg1-/- Bone Marrow." *Arteriosclerosis, Thrombosis, and Vascular Biology* 26 (10): 2308–15.

163. Randolph, Haley E., Zepeng Mu, Jessica K. Fiege, Beth K. Thielen, Jean-Christophe Grenier, Mari S. Cobb, Julie G. Hussin, Yang I. Li, Ryan A. Langlois, and Luis B. Barreiro. 2020. "Single-Cell RNA-Sequencing Reveals Pervasive but Highly Cell Type-Specific Genetic Ancestry Effects on the Response to Viral Infection." *BioRxiv*. https://doi.org/10.1101/2020.12.21.423830.

164. Rastogi, Chaitanya, H. Tomas Rube, Judith F. Kribelbauer, Justin Crocker, Ryan E. Loker, Gabriella D. Martini, Oleg Laptenko, et al. 2018. "Accurate and Sensitive Quantification of Protein-DNA Binding Affinity." *Proceedings of the National Academy of Sciences of the United States of America* 115 (16): E3692–3701.

165. Riordan, J. R., J. M. Rommens, B. Kerem, N. Alon, R. Rozmahel, Z. Grzelczak, J. Zielenski, S. Lok, N. Plavsic, and J. L. Chou. 1989. "Identification of the Cystic Fibrosis Gene: Cloning and Characterization of Complementary DNA." *Science* 245 (4922): 1066–73.

166. Roadmap Epigenomics Consortium, Anshul Kundaje, Wouter Meuleman, Jason Ernst, Misha Bilenky, Angela Yen, Alireza Heravi-Moussavi, et al. 2015. "Integrative Analysis of 111 Reference Human Epigenomes." *Nature* 518 (7539): 317–30.

167. Robins, Chloe, Yue Liu, Wen Fan, Duc M. Duong, Jacob Meigs, Nadia V. Harerimana, Ekaterina S. Gerasimov, et al. 2021. "Genetic Control of the Human Brain Proteome." *American Journal of Human Genetics* 108 (3): 400–410.

168. Robinson, James T., Helga Thorvaldsdóttir, Wendy Winckler, Mitchell Guttman, Eric S. Lander, Gad Getz, and Jill P. Mesirov. 2011. "Integrative Genomics Viewer." *Nature Biotechnology* 29 (1): 24–26.

169. Rommens, J. M., M. C. Iannuzzi, B. Kerem, M. L. Drumm, G. Melmer, M. Dean, R. Rozmahel, J. L. Cole, D. Kennedy, and N. Hidaka. 1989. "Identification of the Cystic Fibrosis Gene: Chromosome Walking and Jumping." *Science* 245 (4922): 1059–65.

170. Sarkar, Abhishek K., Po-Yuan Tung, John D. Blischak, Jonathan E. Burnett, Yang I. Li, Matthew Stephens, and Yoav Gilad. 2019. "Discovery and Characterization of Variance QTLs in Human Induced Pluripotent Stem Cells." *PLoS Genetics* 15 (4): e1008045.

171. Schmiedel, Benjamin J., Divya Singh, Ariel Madrigal, Alan G. Valdovino-Gonzalez, Brandie M. White, Jose Zapardiel-Gonzalo, Brendan Ha, et al. 2018. "Impact of Genetic Polymorphisms on Human Immune Cell Gene Expression." *Cell* 175 (6): 1701-1715.e16.

172. Schmiedel, Benjamin Joachim, Grégory Seumois, Daniela Samaniego-Castruita, Justin Cayford, Veronique Schulten, Lukas Chavez, Ferhat Ay, Alessandro Sette, Bjoern Peters, and Pandurangan Vijayanand. 2016. "17q21 Asthma-Risk Variants Switch CTCF Binding and Regulate IL-2 Production by T Cells." *Nature Communications* 7 (November): 13426.

173. Schork, Nicholas J., Sarah S. Murray, Kelly A. Frazer, and Eric J. Topol. 2009. "Common vs. Rare Allele Hypotheses for Complex Diseases." *Current Opinion in Genetics & Development* 19 (3): 212–19.

174. Schunkert, Heribert, Inke R. König, Sekar Kathiresan, Muredach P. Reilly, Themistocles L. Assimes, Hilma Holm, Michael Preuss, et al. 2011. "Large-Scale Association Analysis Identifies 13 New Susceptibility Loci for Coronary Artery Disease." *Nature Genetics* 43 (4): 333–38.

175. Seifert, Leon Louis, Clara Si, Debjani Saha, Mohammad Sadic, Maren de Vries, Sarah Ballentine, Aaron Briley, et al. 2019. "The ETS Transcription Factor ELF1 Regulates a Broadly Antiviral Program Distinct from the Type I Interferon Response." *PLoS Pathogens* 15 (11): e1007634.

176. Simon, Ruth, Christoph Wiegreffe, and Stefan Britsch. 2020. "Bcl11 Transcription Factors Regulate Cortical Development and Function." *Frontiers in Molecular Neuroscience* 13 (April): 51.

177. Slattery, Matthew, Todd Riley, Peng Liu, Namiko Abe, Pilar Gomez-Alcala, Iris Dror, Tianyin Zhou, et al. 2011. "Cofactor Binding Evokes Latent Differences in DNA Binding Specificity between Hox Proteins." *Cell* 147 (6): 1270–82.

178. Smemo, Scott, Juan J. Tena, Kyoung-Han Kim, Eric R. Gamazon, Noboru J. Sakabe, Carlos Gómez-Marín, Ivy Aneas, et al. 2014. "Obesity-Associated Variants within FTO Form Long-Range Functional Connections with IRX3." *Nature* 507 (7492): 371–75.

179. Smirnov, Denis A., Lauren Brady, Krzysztof Halasa, Michael Morley, Sonia Solomon, and Vivian G. Cheung. 2012. "Genetic Variation in Radiation-Induced Cell Death." *Genome Research* 22 (2): 332–39.

180. Sobreira, Débora R., Amelia C. Joslin, Qi Zhang, Iain Williamson, Grace T. Hansen, Kathryn M. Farris, Noboru J. Sakabe, et al. 2021. "Extensive Pleiotropism and Allelic Heterogeneity Mediate Metabolic Effects of IRX3 and IRX5." *Science* 372 (6546): 1085–91.

181. Stegle, Oliver, Leopold Parts, Richard Durbin, and John Winn. 2010. "A Bayesian Framework to Account for Complex Non-Genetic Factors in Gene Expression Levels Greatly Increases Power in EQTL Studies." *PLoS Computational Biology* 6 (5): e1000770.

182. Stegle, Oliver, Leopold Parts, Matias Piipari, John Winn, and Richard Durbin. 2012. "Using Probabilistic Estimation of Expression Residuals (PEER) to Obtain Increased Power and Interpretability of Gene Expression Analyses." *Nature Protocols* 7 (3): 500–507.

183. Stranger, Barbara E., Alexandra C. Nica, Matthew S. Forrest, Antigone Dimas, Christine P. Bird, Claude Beazley, Catherine E. Ingle, et al. 2007. "Population Genomics of Human Gene Expression." *Nature Genetics* 39 (10): 1217–24.

184. Strober, B. J., R. Elorbany, K. Rhodes, N. Krishnan, K. Tayeb, A. Battle, and Y. Gilad. 2019. "Dynamic Genetic Regulation of Gene Expression during Cellular Differentiation." *Science* 364 (6447): 1287–90.

185. Stunnenberg, Hendrik G., The International Human Epigenome Consortium, and Martin Hirst. 2016. "The International Human Epigenome Consortium: A Blueprint for Scientific Collaboration and Discovery." *Cell* 167 (5): 1145–49.

186. Su, Yan Ru, Dwayne E. Dove, Amy S. Major, Alyssa H. Hasty, Branden Boone, Macrae F. Linton, and Sergio Fazio. 2005. "Reduced ABCA1-Mediated Cholesterol Efflux and Accelerated Atherosclerosis in Apolipoprotein E-Deficient Mice Lacking Macrophage-Derived ACAT1." *Circulation* 111 (18): 2373–81.

187. Tagore, Mohita, Michael J. McAndrew, Alison Gjidoda, and Monique Floer. 2015. "The Lineage-Specific Transcription Factor PU.1 Prevents Polycomb-Mediated Heterochromatin Formation at Macrophage-Specific Genes." *Molecular and Cellular Biology* 35 (15): 2610–25.

188. Taniguchi, Tadatsugu, Kouetsu Ogasawara, Akinori Takaoka, and Nobuyuki Tanaka. 2001. "IRF Family of Transcription Factors as Regulators of Host Defense." *Annual Review of Immunology* 19 (1): 623–55.

189. Taylor, D. Leland, David A. Knowles, Laura J. Scott, Andrea H. Ramirez, Francesco Paolo Casale, Brooke N. Wolford, Li Guan, et al. 2018. "Interactions between Genetic Variation and Cellular Environment in Skeletal Muscle Gene Expression." *PloS One* 13 (4): e0195788-17.

190. Taylor-Weiner, Amaro, François Aguet, Nicholas J. Haradhvala, Sager Gosai, Shankara Anand, Jaegil Kim, Kristin Ardlie, Eliezer M. Van Allen, and Gad Getz. 2019. "Scaling Computational Genomics to Millions of Individuals with GPUs." *Genome Biology* 20 (1): 228.

191. Tehranchi, Ashley K., Marsha Myrthil, Trevor Martin, Brian L. Hie, David Golan, and Hunter B. Fraser. 2016. "Pooled ChIP-Seq Links Variation in Transcription Factor Binding to Complex Disease Risk." *Cell* 165 (3): 730–41.

192. Tuerk, C., and L. Gold. 1990. "Systematic Evolution of Ligands by Exponential Enrichment: RNA Ligands to Bacteriophage T4 DNA Polymerase." *Science* 249 (4968): 505–10.

193. Tushev, Georgi, Caspar Glock, Maximilian Heumüller, Anne Biever, Marko Jovanovic, and Erin M. Schuman. 2018. "Alternative 3' UTRs Modify the Localization, Regulatory Potential, Stability, and Plasticity of MRNAs in Neuronal Compartments." *Neuron* 98 (3): 495-511.e6.

194. Urbut, Sarah Margaret, Gao Wang, Peter Carbonetto, and Matthew Stephens. 2019. "Flexible Statistical Methods for Estimating and Testing Effects in Genomic Studies with Multiple Conditions." *Nature Genetics* 51 (January): 187–95.

195. Vejnar, Charles E., Mario Abdel Messih, Carter M. Takacs, Valeria Yartseva, Panos Oikonomou, Romain Christiano, Marlon Stoeckius, et al. 2019. "Genome Wide Analysis of 3' UTR Sequence Elements and Proteins Regulating MRNA Stability during Maternal-to-Zygotic Transition in Zebrafish." *Genome Research* 29 (7): 1100–1114.

196. Wallace, Chris. 2020. "Eliciting Priors and Relaxing the Single Causal Variant Assumption in Colocalisation Analyses." *PLoS Genetics* 16 (4): e1008720.

197. Wang, Xinchen, and David B. Goldstein. 2020. "Enhancer Domains Predict Gene Pathogenicity and Inform Gene Discovery in Complex Disease." *American Journal of Human Genetics* 106 (2): 215–33.

198. Ward, Michelle C., Nicholas E. Banovich, Abhishek Sarkar, Matthew Stephens, and Yoav Gilad. 2020. "Dynamic Effects of Genetic Variation on Gene Expression Revealed Following Hypoxic Stress in Cardiomyocytes." *BioRxiv*. http://biorxiv.org/lookup/doi/10.1101/2020.03.28.012823.

199. Waszak, Sebastian M., Olivier Delaneau, Andreas R. Gschwind, Helena Kilpinen, Sunil K. Raghav, Robert M. Witwicki, Andrea Orioli, et al. 2015. "Population Variation and Genetic Control of Modular Chromatin Architecture in Humans." *Cell* 162 (5): 1039–50.

200. Webb, Thomas R., Jeanette Erdmann, Kathleen E. Stirrups, Nathan O. Stitziel, Nicholas G. D. Masca, Henning Jansen, Stavroula Kanoni, et al. 2017. "Systematic Evaluation of Pleiotropy Identifies 6 Further Loci Associated With Coronary Artery Disease." *Journal of the American College of Cardiology* 69 (7): 823–36.

201. Weissbrod, Omer, Farhad Hormozdiari, Christian Benner, Ran Cui, Jacob Ulirsch, Steven Gazal, Armin P. Schoech, et al. 2020. "Functionally Informed Fine-Mapping and Polygenic Localization of Complex Trait Heritability." *Nature Genetics* 52 (12): 1355–63.

202. Wen, Xiaoquan, Yeji Lee, Francesca Luca, and Roger Pique-Regi. 2016. "Efficient Integrative Multi-SNP Association Analysis via Deterministic Approximation of Posteriors." *American Journal of Human Genetics* 98 (6): 1114–29.

203. Wen, Xiaoquan, Roger Pique-Regi, and Francesca Luca. 2017. "Integrating Molecular QTL Data into Genome-Wide Genetic Association Analysis: Probabilistic Assessment of Enrichment and Colocalization." *PLoS Genetics* 13 (3): e1006646-25.

204. Westra, Harm-Jan, Danny Arends, Tõnu Esko, Marjolein J. Peters, Claudia Schurmann, Katharina Schramm, Johannes Kettunen, et al. 2015. "Cell Specific EQTL Analysis without Sorting Cells." *PLoS Genetics* 11 (5): e1005223.

205. Wet, J. R. de, K. V. Wood, M. DeLuca, D. R. Helinski, and S. Subramani. 1987. "Firefly Luciferase Gene: Structure and Expression in Mammalian Cells." *Molecular and Cellular Biology* 7 (2): 725–37.

206. White, Jon, Daniel I. Swerdlow, David Preiss, Zammy Fairhurst-Hunter, Brendan J. Keating, Folkert W. Asselbergs, Naveed Sattar, Steve E. Humphries, Aroon D. Hingorani, and Michael V. Holmes. 2016. "Association of Lipid Fractions With Risks for Coronary Artery Disease and Diabetes." *JAMA Cardiology* 1 (6): 692–99.

207. Wijst, Monique G. P. van der, Harm Brugge, Dylan H. de Vries, Patrick Deelen, Morris A. Swertz, LifeLines Cohort Study, BIOS Consortium, and Lude Franke. 2018. "Single-Cell RNA Sequencing Identifies Celltype-Specific Cis-EQTLs and Co-Expression QTLs." *Nature Genetics* 50 (4): 493–97.

208. Wild, Philipp S., Tanja Zeller, Arne Schillert, Silke Szymczak, Christoph R. Sinning, Arne Deiseroth, Renate B. Schnabel, et al. 2011. "A Genome-Wide Association Study Identifies LIPA as a Susceptibility Gene for Coronary Artery Disease." *Circulation. Cardiovascular Genetics* 4 (4): 403–12.

209. Willer, Cristen J., Ellen M. Schmidt, Sebanti Sengupta, Gina M. Peloso, Stefan Gustafsson, Stavroula Kanoni, Andrea Ganna, et al. 2013. "Discovery and Refinement of Loci Associated with Lipid Levels." *Nature Genetics* 45 (11): 1274–83.

210. Yang, Jian, S. Hong Lee, Michael E. Goddard, and Peter M. Visscher. 2011. "GCTA: A Tool for Genome-Wide Complex Trait Analysis." *American Journal of Human Genetics* 88 (1): 76–82.

211. Young, Adam M. H., Natsuhiko Kumasaka, Fiona Calvert, Timothy R. Hammond, Andrew Knights, Nikolaos Panousis, Jun Sung Park, et al. 2021. "A Map of Transcriptional Heterogeneity and Regulatory Variation in Human Microglia." *Nature Genetics* 53 (6): 861–68.

212. Yu, Xiao-Hua, Yu-Chang Fu, Da-Wei Zhang, Kai Yin, and Chao-Ke Tang. 2013. "Foam Cells in Atherosclerosis." *Clinica Chimica Acta; International Journal of Clinical Chemistry* 424 (September): 245–52.

213. Zerbino, Daniel R., Steven P. Wilder, Nathan Johnson, Thomas Juettemann, and Paul R. Flicek. 2015. "The Ensembl Regulatory Build." *Genome Biology* 16 (March): 56.

214. Zhang, Hanrui. 2018. "Lysosomal Acid Lipase and Lipid Metabolism: New Mechanisms, New Questions, and New Therapies." *Current Opinion in Lipidology* 29 (3): 218–23.

215. Zhang, Tongwu, Jiyeon Choi, Michael A. Kovacs, Jianxin Shi, Mai Xu, NISC Comparative Sequencing Program, Melanoma Meta-Analysis Consortium, et al. 2018. "Cell-Type-Specific EQTL of Primary Melanocytes Facilitates Identification of Melanoma Susceptibility Genes." *Genome Research* 28 (11): 1621–35.

216. Zhao, Quanyi, Michael Dacre, Trieu Nguyen, Milos Pjanic, Boxiang Liu, Dharini Iyer, Paul Cheng, et al. 2020. "Molecular Mechanisms of Coronary Disease Revealed Using Quantitative Trait Loci for TCF21 Binding, Chromatin Accessibility, and Chromosomal Looping." *Genome Biology* 21 (1): 135.

217. Zhou, Jian, and Olga G. Troyanskaya. 2015. "Predicting Effects of Noncoding Variants with Deep Learning-Based Sequence Model." *Nature Methods* 12 (10): 931–34.

218. Zhu, Dong-Li, Xiao-Feng Chen, Wei-Xin Hu, Shan-Shan Dong, Bing-Jie Lu, Yu Rong, Yi-Xiao Chen, et al. 2018. "Multiple Functional Variants at 13q14 Risk Locus for Osteoporosis Regulate RANKL Expression Through Long-Range Super-Enhancer." *Journal of Bone and Mineral Research: The Official Journal of the American Society for Bone and Mineral Research* 33 (7): 1335–46.

219. Zhu, Zhihong, Zhili Zheng, Futao Zhang, Yang Wu, Maciej Trzaskowski, Robert Maier, Matthew R. Robinson, et al. 2018. "Causal Associations between Risk Factors and

Common Diseases Inferred from GWAS Summary Data." *Nature Communications* 9 (1): 224.

www.ingramcontent.com/pod-product-compliance
Lightning Source LLC
LaVergne TN
LVHW041105150826
845673LV00007B/1931

* 9 7 8 3 3 8 4 2 7 6 0 1 8 *